Counseling Children
with Hearing Impairment
and Their Families

Related Titles of Interest

Language Learning in Children Who Are Deaf and Hard of Hearing: Multiple Pathways
Susan R. Easterbrooks and Sharon K. Baker
ISBN: 0-205-33100-9

Learning American Sign Language
Tom L. Humphries and Carol A. Padden
ISBN: 0-13-528571-2

Learning American Sign Language Video
Tom L. Humphries and Carol A. Padden
ISBN: 0-13-528969-6

Literacy and Deafness: The Development of Reading, Writing, and Literate Thought
Peter V. Paul
ISBN: 0-205-17576-7

Language and Literacy Development in Children Who Are Deaf, Second Edition
Barbara R. Schirmer
ISBN: 0-205-31493-7

Psychological, Social, and Educational Dimensions of Deafness
Barbara R. Schirmer
ISBN: 0-205-17513-9

Best Practices in Educational Interpreting
Brenda Chafin Seal
ISBN: 0-205-26311-9

Counseling the Communicatively Disabled and Their Families: A Manual for Clinicians
George H. Shames
ISBN: 0-205-30799-X

Interviewing and Counseling in Communicative Disorders: Principles and Procedures, Second Edition
Kenneth G. Shipley
ISBN: 0-205-19892-9

Sign Language Interpreting: Its Art and Science
David A. Stewart, Jerome D. Schein, Brenda E. Cartwright
ISBN: 0-205-27540-0

Teaching Deaf and Hard of Hearing Students: Content, Strategies and Curriculum
David A. Stewart and Thomas N. Kluwin
ISBN: 0-205-30768-X

For further information on these and other related titles, contact:

College Division
Allyn and Bacon, Inc.
75 Arlington Street
Boston, MA 02116
www.ablongman.com

Counseling Children with Hearing Impairment and Their Families

Kristina M. English

Duquesne University

Allyn and Bacon

Boston • London • Toronto • Sydney • Tokyo • Singapore

Executive Editor and Publisher: *Stephen D. Dragin*
Series Editorial Assistant: *Barbara Strickland*
Manufacturing Buyer: *Chris Marson*
Marketing Manager: *Stephen Smith*
Cover Designer: *Suzanne Harbison*
Production Coordinator: *Pat Torelli Publishing Services*
Editorial-Production Service: *Chestnut Hill Enterprises, Inc.*
Electronic Composition: *Publisher's Design and Production Services*

Copyright © 2002 by Allyn & Bacon
A Pearson Education Company
75 Arlington Street
Boston, MA 02116

Internet: www.ablongman.com

Library of Congress Cataloging-in-Publication Data

English, Kristina M.
    Counseling children with hearing impairment and their families /
Kristina M. English.
        p. cm.
    Includes bibliographical references and index.
    ISBN 0-205-32144-5
    1. Hearing impaired children—Counseling of.   2. Deaf children—
Counseling of.   3. Parents of deaf children—Counseling of.   I. Title.

HV2391 .E53 2001
362.4'2'86083—dc21

                                                              2001026673

Printed in the United States of America

10   9   8   7   6   5   4   3   2   1   05   04   03   02   01

As always, to Lewis

CONTENTS

4 Basic Counseling Skills: "Keeping the Door Open"   73

5 Completing the Counseling Process: Goals, Plans, and Intervention   103

ACKNOWLEDGMENTS

I owe a debt of gratitude to the families I have met who have taught me so much about what life is like with hearing loss, as well as to the professionals who serve them. Their voices can be heard throughout this book, and I thank them for generously sharing their stories and insights. I also thank my editor, Steve Dragin, for considering the possibility of this book.

In addition, the following reviewers provided insightful comments: Gail D. Chermak, Washington State University; Tanya Sue Enloe, Valdosta State University; James McCartney, California State University—Sacramento; and George H. Shames, University of Pittsburgh.

Counseling Children with Hearing Impairment and Their Families

Introduction to Nonprofessional Counseling

LEARNING OBJECTIVES

Readers of this chapter will be able to:

1. Distinguish between informational and personal adjustment counseling.
2. Give an example of "communication mismatch."
3. Differentiate between psychotherapy and counseling.
4. Describe the differences between professional and nonprofessional counselors.
5. Describe what is meant by "professional boundaries."

What are the consequences of growing up with a hearing loss? One's first answer might be a broad assumption about missing sounds in the environment, such as not hearing music well or not detecting warning sounds. These answers are accurate, but they only hint at a complex chain of events. Ultimately, the most significant effect of growing up with a hearing loss is its impact on a child's ability to understand others' words, and to develop one's own words. With even a mild degree of hearing loss, a child's vocabulary may develop at a slower rate, and subtle language rules (for example, when and how to change verb tenses or make plurals) are not as easily learned. Children with more severe hearing loss can have even more severe language delays. When language development is delayed, verbal interactions with parents and siblings and the world at large can be difficult and confusing, and relationships can become strained or superficial. When a child is limited in his or her ability in telling a parent about being upset over having to share a toy, that child will feel frustrated, isolated, and mis-understood. When a child asks a new friend how to play an unfamil-iar game, but then doesn't understand the answer, he or she may feel embarrassed and pretend to understand, rather than take the chance that the new friend will think poorly of him or her. The "costs of bluffing" (stress, doubt, and so on) can be stronger than the rewards of socialization, and may discourage a child from interacting with others.

These negative feelings can also contribute to a diminished sense of self-worth—and because of communication limitations, children with hearing loss may have delayed skills in expressing those feelings. They also may not have many people to talk to about how to handle these difficulties.

Growing up with hearing loss, then, not only can result in a broad range of language delays, but also concomitant personal and interper-sonal difficulties. Many types of professionals—educators, audio-logists, speech-language pathologists, school nurses, sign language interpreters, classroom aides—well understand these consequences of growing up with a hearing loss. Because they work with deaf and hard-of-hearing children on a daily basis, they observe social and emo-tional difficulties first-hand, as the following case study depicts:

Case Study: Fatima

In one large school district in a suburban area, the level of audiology services was generally determined by degree of loss: the more severe the hearing loss, the more often the audiologist visited the child. Fatima had a moderate to severe loss, so the audiologist had been checking on her every two weeks since she had started preschool. She was cur-rently attending her neighborhood school, and was the only child en-rolled who had a hearing impairment.

A few months after she had begun fifth grade, the audiologist began to wonder if Fatima was changing somehow: was she losing weight? Did she seem unusually subdued? She was a naturally quiet child, so it was hard to be sure. The audiologist mentioned it to the teacher and the SLP, but since these professionals saw Fatima every day, they were not sure they were seeing any changes; they agreed to keep their eyes open. The following day they both saw Fatima arrive at school in a coat they recognized from the previous year. They immediately saw that not only had Fatima *not* outgrown the coat, it seemed like it had become three sizes too big. Clearly Fatima was losing weight.

Observing a change in behavior, health, or attitude, or identifying a chronic state of unhappiness or maladjustment, is only the first step in helping. However, many professionals feel ill-equipped to do more, that is, to provide direct counseling support. Such hesitancy is not unexpected, since counseling usually is not part of one's background. For example, counseling is included in only 12 percent of the graduate training programs for speech-language pathologists and audiologists (Culpepper, Mendel, & McCarthy, 1994; McCarthy, Culpepper, & Lucks, 1986). When coursework is offered, it will typically describe a range of difficulties observed with respect to self-image, social and interpersonal adjustment, and psychological and emotional health (to be discussed in Chapter 2). However, actual skills needed to support children may not be included. In other words, audiologists and other professionals **know about** psychosocial problems of hearing loss, but many lack the **know-how**—that is, the necessary skills—to help with these problems.

Therefore, an initial reaction to Fatima's situation might be to refer her to a professional counselor. Grunblatt and Daar (1994) describe a program that might be considered a "gold standard" for counseling services: an educational audiologist would provide a series of informational sessions covering topics such as anatomy of the ear, hearing aid use, and audiogram interpretation, and then conclude with an open-ended session to answer children's questions. If their questions seemed to be concerned about personal adjustment issues (for example, "Will I hear when I grow up?" or "Other kids tease me when I don't hear them"), children would be referred to an on-site counselor with expertise in hearing loss and its effects on children's psychological, social, and emotional well-being.

Unfortunately, this type of program is not commonly available, and in fact could be described as rare. Few schools have this kind of support to address adequately the emotional health of children with hearing loss. Therefore, to **know about** psychosocial problems related to hearing loss probably is not enough. The shortage of professional counseling support is good reason for all professionals to consider developing some **know-how**, some basic "nonprofessional" counseling skills (to be described), as a way to strengthen their "safety net" for children with hearing loss.

The "safety net" metaphor is commonly used to describe the array of services made available to children who are deaf and hard of hearing. We would no sooner have children race across a tightrope without a net (Figure 1.1) than we would educate them without these "strands" within our system of service delivery:

- Management of amplification
- Adapted curriculum
- Controlled classroom acoustics
- Interpreters and notetakers
- Socialization opportunities
- Personal/interpersonal counseling support

For our purposes, the "strand" of greatest concern is adequate counseling support. Without it, it is fair to say that our safety net is

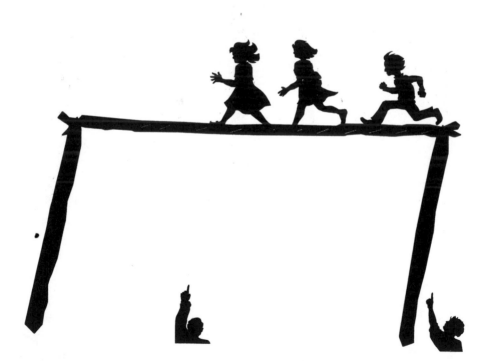

FIGURE 1.1   Improving the safety net for children with hearing loss

flawed, and Chapter 2 will demonstrate some of the reasons why counseling support needs to be "woven" into existing services.

What Do We Mean by Counseling?

Counseling is usually narrowly perceived as "explaining": a professional talks while a patient or student listens. Almost every professional is a "good explainer": school nurses explain how to prevent spreading infections, audiologists clearly explain hearing aid care, SLPs successfully explain techniques in speech production, administrators explain parents' legal rights. A teacher's entire career consists of explaining concepts and vocabulary and directions to follow. Because the purpose of these interactions is to convey information, it can be described as **informational counseling** and is an essential component of a professional's relationship with a child. An example of informational counseling is described in a study by Von Almen and Blair (1989), who developed and tested a comprehension program to teach children how to understand their audiograms and how to care for their amplifications systems. Informational counseling is also the intent of two curricula specifically developed for elementary school children (Marttila & Mills, 1994) and for high school students (English, 1997) with hearing impairment.

One of the characteristics of informational counseling is the direction of conversation: these kinds of exchanges represent a "one-way street" in communication. Since only one person can talk at a time, the majority of that "talk time" is dominated by the professional, while the child listens and works to learn the information conveyed.

Learning is only one aspect of a child's life, of course, and we know that another aspect—one's emotional state—has a direct effect on a child's readiness to learn. A child who is upset, anxious, or worried is at high risk for poor academic performance (Goleman, 1995). But how is a professional to know if a problem exists in a child's life? A child with hearing loss is probably not going to ask for guidance voluntarily if he or she has little experience in self-expression. Instead, the child's "call for help" will more likely be demonstrated by disruptive or troublesome behaviors, which then attract professionals' notice.

When these behaviors occur, it is imperative to recognize **the limitations of informational** counseling, since now we are not interested in explaining technical material or course content. Conversation by necessity now moves into the "realm of the personal." However, it is hard for many professionals to refrain from continuing to provide information, or even to notice that it was not requested. For example, imagine this exchange between a 16 year old student and his teacher:

> **STUDENT:**   I've decided not to wear those hearing aids any more. They make me look ugly and stupid.
>
> **TEACHER:**   But without your hearing aids, you won't hear your teachers and you'll fail your classes.

The student was describing **how he felt** about wearing hearing aids—an affective statement—but the teacher did not respond to those feelings. Instead, the teacher **responded with information** or at least an informed opinion, which the student did not ask for. In fact, the student didn't ask for anything, advice or otherwise, but simply expressed a decision based on feelings. There was more on his mind, but the response from the teacher inadvertently set up a barrier that prevented him from expressing it. Figure 1.2 depicts how such a conversation can be working at cross-purposes: the child is trying to take the conversation in one direction, but the adult is pushing it in another direction.

One can anticipate the trajectory of this conversation along a predictable course: the student will hold fast to his position and the teacher will keep trying to talk him out of it—while the heart of the problem remains unaddressed. These two speakers are not traveling together in the same direction, so communication and understanding will be limited.

This "communication mismatch"—that is, responding to an affective comment with an informational response—may be a common barrier between persons with hearing loss and the professionals who serve them. Studies have found a strong tendency for audiologists to provide informational or content-based responses to affective statements (English, Mendel, Rojeski, & Hornak, 1999; English, Rojeski, & Branham, 2000). For example, to the hypothetical and highly emotional statement: "My family says my daughter is deaf because I worked until the last week of pregnancy," most audiologists in these studies (prior to a course in counseling) did not hear the guilt and grief being expressed, and instead responded with information, along these lines: "There are no studies to prove this, you can rest assured there is no reason to believe it." Ultimately, of course, this information must eventually be conveyed, but this informational response, **at this moment**, does not help

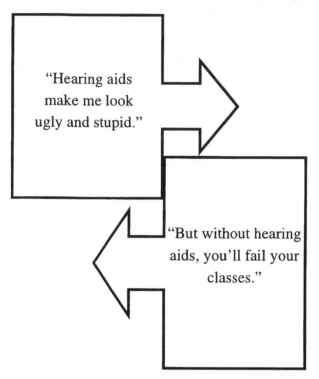

FIGURE 1.2   Mismatching our responses to what we hear

because it does not react to the immediate affective concerns presented. A person's feelings and attitudes generally are not changed by the presentation by a rational argument alone.

When information is not the issue, providing information does not help much—in fact, it may hinder the opportunity to help. A person expressing his or her feelings not only does not register the information being offered, but also feels that he or she is not being understood. Another approach, called **personal adjustment counseling**, attempts to match an affective statement with an affective response—that is, a response that lets a parent or child know that the affect or feeling was heard, and that the listener is attending carefully to that feeling. Instead of the "one-way street" of communication found in informational counseling, personal adjustment counseling uses an "open-ended" approach, which requires that a professional do two very difficult things: (1) stop talking, and (2) listen, or more accurately, listen *effectively*. The ability to "listen effectively" entails two deceivingly simple skills: "opening the door" to conversation, and "keeping the door open" by allowing the child to move the conversation forward as he or she chooses. These skills will be fully explained in Chapters 3 and 4, but for now, let's consider a different version of the previous exchange:

> **STUDENT:**   I've decided not to wear those hearing aids any more. They make me look ugly and stupid.
>
> **TEACHER:**   That's a really big decision.

This deceptively simple response actually accomplishes a great deal. Being neutral and nondirective, it indicates that the teacher (1) heard and understood that the student feels unattractive with hearing aids, (2) acknowledges that this is important to the student, (3) is not judging the child's decision, and (4) is available to hear more if the student wants to provide more. Figure 1.3 depicts a conversation traveling in the same direction, focused on the same concern.

Some writers prefer the term "guidance" to informational counseling (Shipley, 1997), while others call personal adjustment counseling "emotional support counseling" (Clark, 1994). Whichever terms are used, it cannot be stressed enough that we need to have the differences between the two types of counseling clear in our minds, for we cannot expect to provide an appropriate response to a child when we do not recognize the nature of the comment or question: that is, are they asking for information or personal support? Once we know, our responses can have a better chance of being in sync with the child's comments, and what will develop will be a successful "meeting of the minds" (informational counseling) or a successful "heart-to-heart" (personal adjustment counseling). Our goal throughout is to avoid the mismatch problems of a "heart-to-brain" miscommunication (Figure 1.4).

The Counseling Process

When we perceive the need for personal adjustment counseling, we can follow a process established by the counseling profession (Egan, 1998):

☐ Help children tell their story
☐ Help them clarify their problem
☐ Help them challenge themselves to solve the problem

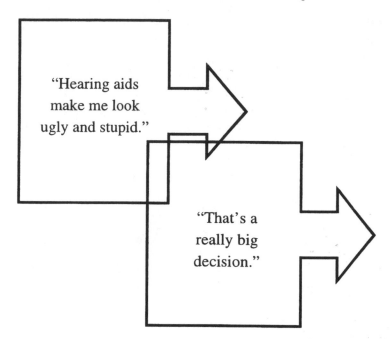

FIGURE 1.3   Matching our responses to what we hear

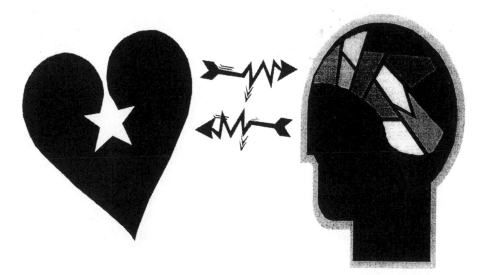

FIGURE 1.4   "Heart-to-brain" or "brain-to-heart" communications are not effective

☐ Help them set a goal
☐ Help them develop an action plan
☐ Observe as they implement the plan
☐ Help them evaluate the plan (Did it accomplish their goal or is more consideration needed? Did a new goal present itself? If so, the process of developing/implementing/evaluating an action plan starts again)

These steps will be fully developed throughout this book. The first step, helping a child tell his or her story, is the sole topic of Chapter 3. Chapter 4 will describe how to help children clarify their problems and challenge themselves to solve them, and Chapter 5 describes the implementation of the four remaining steps.

Is Personal Adjustment Counseling Part of Our Scope of Practice?

Before we go any further, it is likely that the reader is wondering if personal adjustment counseling is an appropriate activity for professionals not formally trained in counseling. The question is a legitimate one, and the answer is yes—as long as two caveats are honored: (1) we remember the differences between professional and nonprofessional counseling, and (2) we respect professional boundaries.

Professional versus Nonprofessional Counseling

Professional counseling is a relatively well-known process today, whereby mental health professionals (such as psychiatrists, psychologists, and social workers) use their professional training to help clients find ways to solve pervasive life problems. Psychotherapy helps patients explore unconscious behavior patterns in order to alter ways of relating and functioning by examining and challenging personal history, and by analyzing the meanings of one's responses (Cormier & Hackney, 1999; Crowe, 1997b; Stone & Olswang, 1989). Shames (2000) describes the differences between psychotherapy and counseling this way:

> The most significant differences are that psychotherapy attempts to restructure the personality, especially in terms of a particular theoretical orientation about the nature and dynamics of personality. Psychother-

apy generally views the patient as being ill and, as a result, searches for the cause or etiology of a person's problems. The person' s overall history, family relationships, and the reliving of childhood trauma are viewed as keys to resolution. . . .

Counseling, by contrast, deals with the present, with here-and-now strategies for coping with life, decision making, and current problems . . . Instead of a medical illness approach, a learning model is employed whereby the counselor helps clients to become aware of themselves, of what they believe and feel, and how these things affect what they do and how they interact with society . . . The overlap between counseling and psychotherapy comes primarily from the tactics used during clinical interviews, and not from their underlying theoretical dynamics or goals. (pp. 6–7)

In other words, while psychotherapy attempts to affect major personality changes, counseling focuses on relatively minor personal adjustments to situations by helping a person understand his or her feelings and engage in problem solving.

Nonprofessional counseling may not be as familiar a concept, but it occurs routinely: a financial planner will counsel on tax problems, a teacher will counsel on test-taking strategies, an audiologist will counsel on hearing conservation, and so on (Kennedy & Charles, 1989). These examples all involve informational counseling, but all professionals on occasion will work with clients or students facing emotional crises as well (for example, the stress associated with financial risk, or the despair and discouragement from failing an important exam). When the emotional crisis is related to the professional's specialty, **nonprofessional personal adjustment counseling** can be an invaluable support.

Professional Boundaries

Stone and Olswang (1989) caution professionals to recognize their limits or boundaries as nonprofessional counselors. They define boundaries as a way to define relationships with rules that clarify the roles and functions of individuals in the relationship.

For adults, these "rules" are often unspoken understandings of conventional behavior. For example, a group of strangers sitting together in an auditorium, waiting for a lecture to begin, may engage in conversations of the most impersonal kind, such as comparisons of parking or traffic problems or observations on room temperature. If a person discloses details of his or her life that exceed the unspoken limits of sharing personal information, the listener will feel uncomfortable and distance him- or herself at least psychologically if not literally from the speaker, thereby expressing a "rule" of expected behavior.

Between adults and children, the rules may be either spoken or unspoken, since the socialization process includes explicit instructions on how to interact with adults. For example, teachers will establish a boundary with children by introducing themselves with titles like Ms., Mr., or Dr., and children will be corrected if they attempt to use first names.

Counseling boundaries also involve attending to the comfort level of the interaction. If the content or the type of interaction brings on a "gut feeling" or a "red flag" of inappropriateness, the boundaries of counseling are being challenged and need to be respected. A sense of inappropriateness could apply either to the *content* of the interaction (feelings, attitudes, problems related to hearing loss), or to the *style* of the interaction (e.g., too intimate for the situation, or overly intense or threatening). Professionals should respect their own reactions and refer to professional counselors if they feel uncomfortable. It is important not to see this as failure but as taking the next vital step in making sure the individual gets the right help (Clark, 1999).

Counseling boundaries are drawn along "lines of expertise." It is not expected and in fact is inappropriate for nonprofessional counselors to attempt to help with marital problems, substance abuse, financial difficulties, domestic violence, clinical depression, and so on. When these concerns arise, we must refer to professional counselors and protect our boundaries with great care. Referral processes are described in detail in Chapter 5.

Case Study: Martin

"Ms. D" was a school speech-language pathologist newly assigned to Metro School. Among the children on her new caseload was Martin, a 10-year-old with a cochlear implant. Ms. D. was interested in seeing how Martin was doing in his mainstream classroom, so she arranged for a time with his teacher to observe him during several activities. The teacher reported that Martin was a strong student, very conscientious in his studies, "a real bookworm."

Ms. D. came to class on a Friday morning and sat in the back of the room. She observed what the teacher had described: Martin did read a great deal, even when other children were working together on a paper mache map or developing the classroom newsletter. While these children worked, Ms. D. heard frequent mention of a birthday party being held that weekend. From the sound of it, the entire class was attending.

Ms. D. took a moment to introduce herself to Martin, and asked about the book he was reading. Before leaving, she said to him, "Have fun at that birthday party tomorrow." His eyes widened and he shook his head, then quickly returned to his book. Ms. D. wondered, was he uncomfortable with social activities? She asked the teacher on the way out, "Do you know why Martin isn't going to the party tomorrow?" The teacher nodded and said softly, "He wasn't invited. He and one other boy were not included. Martin hasn't been invited to a party yet—he hasn't made any friends."

Is it our concern that Martin is not making friends? Do professionals see social skills and friendship development as their responsibility? This question has no definitive answer, since academics naturally get first priority in school settings, and it is frequently assumed that social development "takes care of itself."

However, some would argue that addressing a child's personal adjustment concerns is not only part of one's scope of practice, but is actually among its most important components (Hartup, 1996). For instance, Sanders (1993) is emphatic in stating, "If there were to be one criterion by which the effectiveness of a program of intervention for hearing impaired children might be assessed, it would be the child's personal adjustment . . . It is the impact of the communication/learning handicap on the child's sense of self-worth and well-being that most severely limits the quality of his life" (p. 373).

Case Study: Curtis

Curtis is a sophomore in high school, has a moderate hearing loss, and is new to the area. He figured an easy way to make friends would be through sports, in which he has always excelled. He tried out for the track team, and was uncomfortably surprised that most of the students were much better runners than he was used to, so he was happy to make junior varsity. He was a little worried, though, about his ability to compete with so many strong athletes.

The week after tryouts, Curtis was rushing from math to science class. As always, the halls were noisy with lockers slamming and people yelling. Someone called from behind, "Hey, Turtle, are you going to practice today?" He assumed this was a reference to his relatively slow running; he felt humiliated and became so upset that he turned around and, almost before he knew it, shoved a student against the wall with his shoulder. "Don't call me turtle," he yelled. The student who had addressed him looked angry but also confused: "What are you talking about?" A third student nearby figured it out: "He said 'hey Curt,' not 'hey turtle.' What are you all worked up about? You need to lighten up." Curtis was mortified. He mumbled, "Sorry," and slipped away fast, and decided dropping out of track was preferable to facing that student again.

Our Challenge: To Strengthen Our "Safety Net" with Counseling Support

Why is 11 year old Fatima losing weight? Why is Martin not included in social events? Why did Curtis automatically assume an insult was intended in that exchange? Each child described here would benefit from talking to someone who understood their circumstances. The idea of a safety net was mentioned before, and indeed children do have a partial net already available to them. In an ideal world, they have families who love them, teachers who work hard for them, friends who enjoy their company, professional counselors to talk to, and several other supports as well. Many children do not have so ideal a world, so there can be big gaps in their net. This book is designed to give professionals some basic skills in counseling to help them strengthen the net they hold for the children they serve.

How This Book is Organized

This book is arranged to approximate the steps that counseling students go through as they master basic counseling skills (Egan, 1998). These steps are as follows:

1. Developing cognitive understanding, or "knowing" basic theories and rationales, and pertinent research literature. In Chapter 2, we will start at this first step, by spending considerable time reviewing the research so that we have the essential cognitive understanding of the psychosocial and emotional concerns among children with hearing loss. However, it was earlier recognized

that "knowing is not enough"; therefore, help will be provided to work our way through the remaining steps:

2. Clarification (getting questions answered, confusions cleared up)
3. Modeling (a description of how an interaction should be handled)
4. Written exercises ("practicing in private")
5. Practice
6. Feedback

These five learning steps are incorporated in the "Learning Activities" at the end of Chapters 1 through 5. It will be noted that most activities involve the cooperation and interaction with a learning partner. It is a given that one cannot acquire counseling skills independently; it requires practice and interaction, and ultimately, learning-by-doing.

The final step in learning the counseling process is:

7. Evaluation of the learning experience. To help the reader complete at least one full cycle of learning counseling skills, a self-evaluation process is presented in Chapter 6.

Chapter Summary

- Few children with hearing loss have access to professional counseling support in their school settings. Nonprofessional counselors can improve coverage as these children (and their parents) face challenges in their psychosocial and emotional development.
- Nonprofessional counseling skills involve knowing when to convey information and knowing when to provide support to personal adjustment concerns.
- Professional boundaries determine when a referral to a professional counselor is warranted.

Learning Activities

Clarification Activities

Explain to a learning partner the differences between:

- Psychotherapy and counseling
- Professional and nonprofessional counseling
- Informational counseling and personal adjustment counseling

With a learning partner or small group, brainstorm ten possible reasons to account for:

- Fatima's weight loss
- Martin's isolation
- Curtis's overreaction

Modeling Activity

Identify a person in your environment whom you consider to be an effective counselor or at least a gifted listener. Obtain permission to observe him or her for one hour or more while interacting with others (without breaching confidentiality concerns).

Writing Activity

Create a list describing this person's characteristics and listening behaviors. Underline those that seem to be unique to this person (attributable mostly to personality), and circle those that appear "teachable" to others.

Practice/Feedback Activity

With a learning partner, discuss insights from the observation and written exercise. Apply what was learned in the written exercise to a role-playing activity. With the partner, take on the parts of the student and adult in the following scenario:

> **STUDENT:** I've decided not to wear those hearing aids any more. They make me look ugly and stupid.
>
> **TEACHER:** That's a really big decision.

Extend the scene by adding at least 5 more exchanges between parties. Then discuss: did the "student" feel listened to? Why or why not? Did the "teacher" struggle with what to say to keep the conversation going? Why or Why not? Was it easy or difficult to translate what was observed and described in writing into action?

2 What We Know: Children with Hearing Loss Are at Risk

LEARNING OBJECTIVES

Readers of this chapter will be able to:

1. Describe self-concept and how external messages influence the development of "self."
2. Describe the effects of hearing loss on the development of self-concept.
3. Define the "hearing aid effect."
4. Identify a range of concerns in the psychosocial and emotional development of children who have hearing impairment.

This chapter will provide highlights of the research available on the emotional, social, and psychological development of children with hearing loss. The impact of hearing loss on a child's family also briefly will be considered. While much of what we know comes from studies considering only deaf children, no distinction between deaf and hard of hearing children will be made here. Interested readers are referred to "Suggested Readings" at the end of this chapter for resources which look at the unique issues of deafness.

In addition, the information conveyed in this chapter is not meant to imply that all children with hearing loss will experience all the difficulties described herein. No doubt, readers can name many children who are growing up happy, well adjusted, and high achieving. However, as a population, there is reason for professionals to maintain vigilance, and to ask themselves at any given time, "Is the child I see in front of me right now at risk for any of these difficulties?"

Growing Up with Hearing Loss

To Begin At the Beginning: Self-Concept

It has been observed that many children with hearing loss do not have a highly positive perception of themselves. Therefore, a consideration of the development of self-concept is a logical starting point in our consideration of their psychosocial and emotional development.

Although at first it may seem counter-intuitive, the development of self-concept does not come from the self. Rather, it is learned by absorbing the input and feedback and reactions from those around us. Ultimately, self-concept does involve one's own "evaluation of his or her own traits, attitudes, social position and self in general . . . it is the way a person feels and thinks about him or herself" (Warren & Hasenstab, 1986, p. 289). But those first evaluations are "reflected appraisals," received initially and primarily from family members. "As contact continues, the child interprets and finds meaning for him or herself through these appraisals" (p. 292–93).

People in the world around us are not very skilled or even very interested in hiding these appraisals or attitudes; rather, they are likely to wear them on their sleeves. As recipients of those attitudes, we usually notice and care about these attitudes, for few of us are so self-confident as to be utterly uninfluenced by the opinion of others (Byrne, 1996).

However, children are obviously more vulnerable than adults to others' appraisals. They are likely to internalize those appraisals without question, and to allow these attitudes to "define themselves to themselves." Self-concept then is developed through a process of exploration and input, whereby we learn "what is me" and "what is not me." Children are likely to think these thoughts: "I see myself the way you tell me you see me. If you see me as smart or dumb, loved or unlovable, a joy or a burden—this is how I see myself. This is what I will become, or else I will reject and struggle against these attitudes for much of my life." This process has been described as the "circular effect" of self-concept development: receiving input, accepting or rejecting its validity, and then receiving more input about that decision (Combes & Gonzales, 1994; Marsh, 1992).

With age and experience comes some ability to keep others' opinions in balance with one's hard-fought-for self-concept, but developmental psychologists specializing in adulthood and the aging process indicate that the ego is always susceptible at some level to the consideration of "what others think." Since self-concept is learned, it can be also modified or influenced, but not without some pain and effort.

The concern for positive self-concept suffered some bad press in the 1980s and 1990s, when, in the interest of improving academic achievement, some school systems adopted curricula designed to promote positive self-concept or high self-esteem (Branthwaite, 1985; Purkey, 1984; Strein, 1993). The intent was to validate success achieved by hard work, but instead it became watered down as an effort to praise every insignificant act, while avoiding the possibility of hurting the child's feelings. These programs were roundly criticized and quickly abandoned—a regrettable outcome, since these efforts to address negative self-concept were based on sound research showing strong relationships to school absenteeism, drop-out rates, teenage pregnancy, and teen drug use (Goleman, 1995; Rumberger, 1995; Pudlas, 1996). During and beyond school years, negative self-concept is a primary concern among persons seeking professional counseling.

Family as First Shapers of Self-Concept

As primary caregivers, parents are the first shapers of a child's self-concept. If parents feel competent and capable of eventually adjusting to the unexpected presence of a disability in their family, the child is more likely to feel accepted as important, valued, and loved. If parents have ongoing difficulty coping with their child's hearing loss, their child may internalize their reactions as an expression of their limited acceptance or even rejection of him or her.

Following is an example of how a child learns "who I am" from a parent:

Scene: A fast-food restaurant.   An 8-year-old boy stands in line with his mother to buy some hamburgers. A 5 year old girl stares at his bright blue earmolds and tells her own mother in a very loud voice, "That boy put gum in his ears!" Several people turn around to look.

The boy flushes, and looks at his mother, silently checking with her, "How do I react?" Mom smiles, gives a tiny shrug and winks at him, as if to say, "Not this again!" He nods, taking her lead, and shrugs too—they have talked many times about how people are not well-informed about hearing loss, and how they will say things that can be upsetting if one allows.

Mother's message is loud and clear: "This does not embarrass me, you do not embarrass me, I am fine with this event, and you can be fine too." This minor incident would be one in an ongoing series of events where the child gets positive coping messages from the parent as well as an ongoing sense of security and support. "Parents who are sensitive to their children's needs create a 'secure base' for their children. Securely attached [children] use their parents as secure bases from which to explore the world; in doing so, an optimal balance is met between the need for attachment to caregivers and the need to explore the environment" (Pipp-Siegel & Biringen, 2000, p. 238).

However, Warren and Hasenstab (1986) suggest that "Although parents of hearing-impaired children want to do what is best for them, most have difficulty coping with their child's hearing loss" (p. 293). In their roles as "first shapers," such difficulties could inadvertently contribute to a child's negative self-perception. Of course it must be acknowledged that, given the "nature-nurture" debate, it is impossible to attribute one variable as the only shaper of a child's self-concept, and throughout this book, we will operate with the firm belief that parents use their best abilities throughout the challenges they face. Overall, we can consider a child's self-concept as a "work-in-progress," a canvas that is vulnerable to many paint brushes (Figure 2.1).

Parents and Families Have Self-Concepts Too

Early on and often across time, parents do not always have all the skills or personal resources needed to provide influential positive messages. From the moment the diagnosis of hearing loss was made, their lives are different from what they had expected, and the adjustment process cannot be predicted or hurried. Over time, they work their way through the expected self-concept of being parents of a "perfect" child, to the "new reality" of being parents of a child who has a hearing loss, and this process can be harder for some parents than for others. Kricos (2000) writes about professionals' perceptions of parents who are struggling with acceptance:

> Parents in the denial stage may appear to clinicians to be blocking efforts to initiate the intervention program. However, it should be remembered that this initial reaction to the diagnosis may provide a time for parents to search for inner strength and accumulate information. The goal for clinicians during this stage of grieving is to find ways of not merely tolerating parental denial but accepting it, while still offering, to

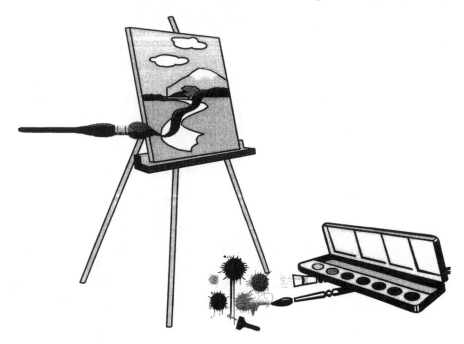

FIGURE 2.1   Self-concept as a vulnerable canvas

the best of their abilities, the services the child needs. Unfortunately, parents who appear to be denying their child's hearing impairment are often perceived by clinicians as foolish and stubborn, when they should be perceived as loving parents who, for the time being, cannot accept the professional's diagnosis of such a severe disability in their child. (p. 279–80)

A parent was once heard to say, "Parents and professionals live in two different time zones: professionals want immediate decisions and immediate action, and express a terrifying sense of urgency. The thing is, parents would rather that time stood still, for at least a little while. The world beneath us has suddenly been jerked out from under us, and we need time to find our footing again." Actively appreciating the need for parents to pace themselves through the adjustment process, while they also look after other ongoing family and employment concerns, should be a high priority for professionals. In Chapter 3, the concept of *positive unconditional regard* will be presented. Readers will be asked to consider this concept with respect to parents as well as to children.

How Families Define Themselves

"Family" has been described by a concept called *family systems theory*, which postulates that circumstances affecting one family member ultimately affect all family members. Whether the circumstance is financial status, lifestyle choices, or the presence of a disability, the entire family, as a system, must adjust to it (Turnbull & Turnbull, 1990).

Family can also be defined by a set of interdependent variables, and it may be helpful to consider these variables when getting to know a child's family:

- *Structure*, or the descriptive elements of the family: number of adults and children, socioeconomic status, education, cultural background, religion, presence or absence of a disability.
- *Resources*, or a family's strengths and coping strategies. Resources include finances but can also include physical and mental health, extended family/community, and religious or spiritual supports. Coping strategies that can provide resources include passive appraisal ("putting a problem on the back burner" until ready to address it); reframing a situation ("At least it's not as bad as leukemia . . ."); or seeking support (spiritual, social, or formal support from agencies). Social support has been found to be an important resource in coping with stress among hearing mothers of children with hearing loss (Calderon & Greenberg, 1999).
- *Interaction*, or how a family deals with events of daily life and accomplishes the "work" of family: providing affection and support, sharing responsibilities, making plans for the future. Family interactions are defined by three characteristics, all of which exist on a continuum and most of which are found near the "average":
  - Attachment (levels of dependence). The continuum for attachment ranges from "enmeshed," where family goals fully subsume individuals' needs, to "disengaged," where members share the same residence but live parallel lives.
  - Adaptability (the ability to adapt to change or stress). The continuum for adaptability ranges from "rigid," where there exists only predetermined roles and no negotiation, to "chaotic," where there are no rules and no consistency at all.
  - Communication, which can range from "closed" where problems are not discussed (as in the movie *Ordinary People*), to "random," where every small and large thing is discussed with equally high levels of emotion.

- *Family functions* as they fulfill the range of family needs: economics, domestic, recreation, self-identify, affection, education, socialization. A primary family function is the emotional support we all expect; however, it has been observed that parents who do not share the same hearing status as their children show lower levels of emotional availability (i.e., emotional openness, emotional communication) than those who do (Jamieson, 1995; Mendel, 1997; Pipp-Siegel & Biringen, 2000). Interactions between parent and child tend to be briefer, more directive, more negative, and more rigid. Less praise is observed. These are consequences of the limited communication between parent and child as a result of the hearing loss, part of a complicated pattern that parents don't always understand until it is pointed out to them.
- *Family life cycle*, which moves from childbearing years to school-age years, adolescence, young adult, post-parental, and aging. Transition through these stages are difficult for most families, but are often not well-defined when a disability is part of family identity.

Understanding family systems is considered an important first step for professionals as they support the family in its ongoing adjustment to hearing loss. The family system means, of course, not only mother and father, but all brothers and sisters and extended family as well. Siblings of children with hearing loss are likely to perceive disproportionate attention to their brother or sister's disability, and resent this while simultaneously experiencing "survivor guilt." As a child not born with a disability, siblings often feel the need to be "extra good" so as not to further upset parents. Their "good work" at school or home may be overlooked by fatigued or distracted parents. Extended family (grandparents, aunts, uncles, and others) are rarely discussed in the research literature, but experience and intuition tell us that they too experience deep grief and conflict when a child is diagnosed with a disability. Different family members cope in different ways, frequently in diametrically opposed ways, and strong differences in opinions on how hearing loss should be managed can add more strain to an already strained system. Professionals are rarely privy to all the tensions that a family is experiencing, and surely would be humbled if they did know.

Our focus shifts now from family systems back to self-concept and how it can be affected by hearing impairment.

Self-Concept and Hearing Impairment

What happens to the development of self-concept when hearing loss is factored in? It appears that children with hearing loss are more likely to have a relatively poor self-concept, most often from resultant communication problems and also from "feeling different" as a hearing aid user (Pudlas, 1996). Some insight is provided by Loeb and Sarigiani (1986), who asked 64 hard-of-hearing children in mainstream settings to respond to questions from the *Children's Self-Concept Scale* (Piers & Harris, 1964), and then compared their answers to children with no disabilities, as well as to children with visual impairment. The 80 questions of this scale give an indication of the extent to which children felt positive about themselves (for example, I have good ideas: Yes or no.)

Regardless of the degree of their hearing loss, children with hearing impairment indicated poorer self-esteem compared to both children with vision impairments and children with no impairments. They expressed relatively more dissatisfaction with how they perceived themselves, most often as feeling less likeable, overly shy and socially isolated (most likely because of their communication difficulties). They also indicated having a hard time making friends, and that often they are not chosen as playmates. Their teachers confirmed these self-perceptions, also describing the children as generally being shy and having problems with peer relationships.

This study also asked children to complete five open-ended statements. The statements were:

> I am happy when_____
> I am sad when _____
> The thing I like most in the world is _____
> The thing I would most like to change is _____
> Because I cannot hear (or see) too well, _____

The responses to the open-ended statements indicated isolation from family and peers. While the majority of children with no hearing loss indicated that they most liked being home with family or with friends, few children with hearing loss so indicated. Rather, they more often reported enjoying playing or being involved in solitary activities. Rather than feeling valued or secure in their families, they tended to describe themselves as unimportant and even as a source of disappointment.

In 1995, Cappelli and colleagues reported additional observations about children with hearing impairment and self-concept. The researchers collected information from 23 children with a range of hearing losses, from ages 6–12, all in oral/aural education programs, as well as from 23 children with no hearing loss, matched by gender and classroom. From a "Self Perception Profile for Children," it was found that children with hearing impairment perceived themselves as less socially accepted than their nonhearing-impaired peers.

The second part of the study demonstrates the "circular effect" of social input to self-esteem and self-concept, described earlier in this chapter. A technique called *sociometrics* was used to determine the social status of all subjects, as indicated by their classmates. Each classmate was asked to use a "likability scale" by naming the three children they would most like to play with (positive nomination), and also the three children they would least like to play with (negative nomination). The outcomes identify children with high or low social status. Children with hearing impairment were nominated less often as friends, and were identified as having low social status from negative nominations 39 percent of the time, while only 5 percent of children without hearing impairment received negative nominations. The degree of hearing loss was not related to these findings. However, it was found that children with hearing loss who did demonstrate higher social status also demonstrated higher self-esteem. In other words, using the "circular effect" model (Figure 2.2), it would appear that the self-perception of being socially accepted helps heighten the sense of self-worth, which then probably enhances social acceptability (since people generally like other people who are confident and secure). The reverse of this circle also seemed to hold true: most children with hearing loss actually rated themselves as even lower in social status than their peers did.

A more recent study (Bess, Dodd-Murphy, & Parker, 1998) asked more than 1,200 children with mild hearing loss to complete a measure called the *COOP Adolescent Chart* (Nelson et al. 1987), which posed questions such as, "During the past month, how often have you felt badly about yourself?" with answers placed on a 5-point scale, from "none of the time" to "all of the time." Overall, children with mild hearing loss exhibited significantly higher dysfunction in the self-esteem subtest

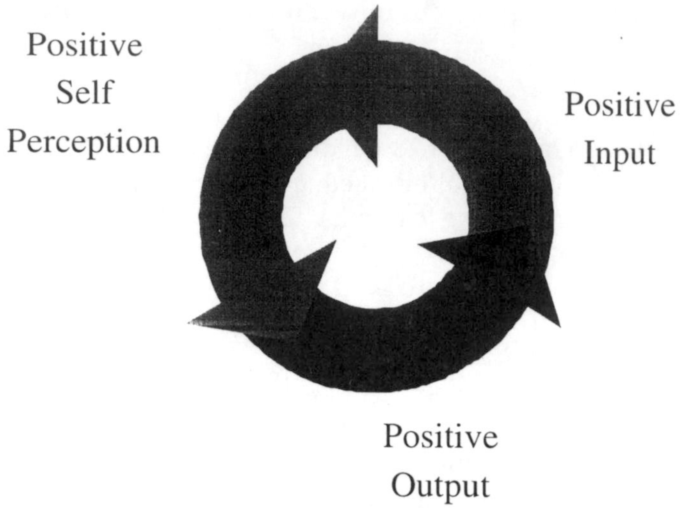

Positive
Self
Perception

Positive
Input

Positive
Output

FIGURE 2.2   The cyclical nature of self-concept development

than children without hearing loss. The researchers concluded that "even mild losses can be associated with increased social and emotional dysfunction among school aged children" (p. 350).

Maxon, Brackett, and van den Berg (1991) asked 41 mainstreamed students with a range of hearing impairment to complete a "Social Awareness Measure" to learn how they would answer to items such as "I help other kids" or "I yell at people." For comparison, 22 children without hearing loss also completed the measure. Results suggests that children with hearing loss saw themselves as less verbally expressive emotionally and less verbally aggressive, even though their verbal communication skills were considered by teachers to be age-appropriate.

We can consider these reports an expression of how one feels as coming from "the self." However, how one feels is also influenced by external or social forces: opinions, attitudes, and reactions from others are powerful influences on our emotional state. As social beings, we care, worry about, and are affected by the positive or negative reactions we receive from those around us. Lapore (1997) writes that ". . . The social environment can moderate or alter the impact of chronic stressors [such as hearing loss] by mitigating or exacerbating people's responses to them" (p. 133). So children have two stressors: (1) They must work through their own emotional reactions to being persons with hearing loss, as well as (2) Decide how much importance to place on social approval and acceptance.

Self-Concept and the "Hearing Aid Effect"

Readers will notice how the discussion on self-concept has begun to shift back and forth between the perceptions of the child and perceptions of others. The two perspectives are intrinsically interdependent, because each directly influences the other. A case in point is the phenomenon known as "the hearing aid effect," a term coined in a study that asked 50 college students with normal hearing to view a set of photographic slides of adolescents, some wearing visible hearing aids and some not (Blood, Blood, & Danhauer, 1977). Viewers were asked to rate each individual in 20 categories of intelligence, capability, attractiveness, and personality. All characteristics were identical except for the presence of hearing aids, yet when the instruments were seen, individuals were given lower scores in almost every category. It appears that the very presence of a hearing aid caused overall negative reactions.

These negative impressions have been replicated in other studies, including one using school-age children as raters (Dengerink & Porter, 1984). This time, 100 fifth- and sixth-grade children were asked to rate photographs of boys of the same age, some wearing hearing aids or glasses. Raters were asked to judge, on a scale from 1 to 6, fifteen characteristics such as "good looking/plain," "productive/nonproductive," and "active/passive." These children gave significantly more negative ratings to the boys wearing hearing aids, although not to those wearing glasses. The authors felt this finding suggested that glasses are socially acceptable but hearing aids are not.

Another version of this study was conducted with preschool children (Riensche, Peterson, & Linden, 1990), using questions such as, "How much do you like this child?" and "How much does this child need help from others?" Preschoolers viewed 12 pictures of same-age peers who wore either a body-style hearing aid or a behind-the-ear instrument, or no aid at all. Interestingly, no differences in responses were measured across the three conditions, leading the researchers to suspect that bias toward hearing aid users does not develop until the early school grades.

Interestingly, when a group of classroom teachers were given this type of exercise, they did not associate any negative attributes to children wearing hearing aids either (Brimacombe, Danhauer, & Mulac, 1983). It cannot be known if results were influenced by an "overcompensation on the part of the teachers to respond in a socially appropriate manner" (p. 133), as the authors suspected, but it has been observed anecdotally that many teachers at least have lower expectations for children with hearing loss.

What do devices like hearing aids and cochlear implants have to do with self-concept? We do not have any controlled studies to tell us what we think we already know: that the appearance of a device on the ear or head not only negatively affects people who see it, but their reaction is likely to be perceived by the hearing aid user. Edwards (1991) reminds us that "The psychosocial aspects of using amplification are often an almost forgotten dynamic in children's acceptance of wearing hearing aids or FM systems. . . . It is the wearing of the device which 'amplifies' the difference between the child with hearing loss and his or her peers" (p. 7).

The interplay between self-concept and others' perceptions was discovered in a study that divided a group of older women, and gave half of them hearing aids to wear (Doggett, Stein, & Gans, 1998). All subjects then interacted with unfamiliar same-age peers who later rated them on attractiveness, friendliness, confidence, and intelligence. The subjects who wore the hearing aids were rated as less confident, friendly, and intelligent than the subjects not wearing hearing aids. The remarkable point about this study is that the raters did not notice the hearing aids, and so were not responding to their appearance! The authors surmised that the subjects wearing hearing aids displayed less confidence, friendliness, and intelligence, projecting a negative self-image to which the raters responded.

If adults are uncomfortable wearing hearing aids, and feel self-conscious about it to the point of projecting a negative self-image, might not children be too? We know that self-concept integrates internal or emotional responses to a situation (such as the generally negative emotional reactions to living with hearing loss), and the external or social feedback from others in our lives (such as the reactions to hearing loss and amplification—also frequently negative). Ignoring the hearing aid effect is akin to ignoring the proverbial elephant standing in the middle of the living room. It would be naive to assume that because children have been using hearing aids for several years, they (and their parents) are not vulnerable to this "hearing aid effect."

"Back to Cases": Fatima

Let us revisit our first case study from Chapter 1. It had been noticed that Fatima was losing weight and becoming withdrawn. What do we know about her self-concept? Might she be losing confidence in herself as she becomes more aware of being the only child in school with a hearing loss? Is she losing the sense of who she is? Is she so unhappy that she is on the verge of clinical depression? How can we find out if we can help her?

Chapters 3 and 4 will attempt to answer that last question, but for now we will move beyond self-concept to other aspects of a child's development. It will be soon become apparent that psychological, social, and emotional development are embedded in self-concept.

Psychosocial Development

Most of this section will address socialization and interpersonal relationships, since nonprofessional counselors by definition are not qualified to provide support to children exhibiting significant psychological difficulties. Comprehensive descriptions of the **psychological development** of children with hearing loss have been developed by other sources, and will only be highlighted here.

These kinds of psychological difficulties have been described by Meadow (1976, 1980), who reported how children with severe to profound hearing loss have been characterized as compulsive, egocentric, and rigid. Deficits in empathy have been described (Bachara, Raphael, & Phelan, 1980), as well as higher than expected levels of anxiety (Harris, Van Zandt, & Rees, 1997), and a condition called "primitive personality" among deaf individuals (McCay, 1996):

> This disorder involves a combination of extreme educational deprivation (usually functional illiteracy), miniscule social input and knowledge, including awareness of appropriate social behavior, immaturity, and a generally psychologically barren life. While not psychotic, individuals with primitive personalities are not able to cope with life in our complex modern society. When the communication handicap of deafness is not dealt with, educationally and psychologically, primitive personality is a frequent result. (p. 237)

While few people with hearing impairment experience a genuinely "extreme deprivation," most do contend with limited input that can result in a reduced repertoire of coping skills. Frustrations and worries that cannot be verbally expressed can escalate into impulse disorder-type behavior or depression. It must be understood that psychological difficulties are not caused by a hearing loss per se, but rather by the language deficits that are concomitant with hearing loss. If these kinds of concerns present themselves, a referral to a qualified psychologist or other counselor is in order.

Less complex but still important difficulties have been observed in the **social development** among children with hearing loss. Because of their delay in developing communication skills, children with hearing loss have fewer opportunities for peer interactions, making it difficult to learn "the social rules governing communication" (Antia & Kreimeyer, 1992, p. 135). Poor and limited communication results in poor social competence. **Social competence** has been described by Greenberg and Kusche (1993) as involving these abilities:

1. Good communication skills
2. The capacity to think independently
3. The capacity for self-direction and self-control
4. Understanding the feelings, motivations, and needs of self and others
5. Flexibility adapting to the needs of a particular situation
6. The ability to tolerate frustration
7. The capacity to tolerate ambivalence in one's feelings and thinking
8. The ability to rely on and be relied on by others
9. Understanding and appreciating one's own culture and values, and those of others
10. Maintaining healthy relationships with others

It would appear that children with hearing loss are at risk in developing these social competencies (Raymond & Matson, 1989; Schum, 1991). For instance, a group of parents of 40 children with hearing impairment completed a questionnaire, and overall indicated that their children had more than typical problems interacting with others and establishing friendships (Davis, Elfenbein, Schum, & Bentler, 1986). The children themselves were interviewed, and 50 percent (N = 20) expressed their own concerns about peers and social relationships. Most children stated they would not mention wearing hearing aids because of "a fear of being teased and embarrassed, and many others reported spending most of their time alone" (p. 60). The researchers wondered if these social problems were typical among most preadolescents, so they conducted the same interview among 58 children without hearing loss. After factoring out the responses from two children who had just moved to a new school, only 12 percent (N = 7) of these children reported having difficulty making friends or getting teased.

Teasing seems to be a pervasive concern. In another study (English, 2001), more than half (59%) of a group of 22 hard of hearing children, ages 8–12, indicated that they got teased about their hearing loss. Responses were obtained by using a scale called the *Children's Peer Relationship (CPR) Scale*. (The *CPR Scale*, described in detail in Chapter 3, was not designed to compare children with and without hearing loss, but rather to "open the door" to a conversation about friends and self-concept.) Only 55 percent of the children in this study agreed with the statement that "Mostly, other kids like me," while the remaining students indicated that "Sometimes other kids don't like me" (27%) or "Other kids don't really like me" (18%). Interestingly, in this study, their classroom teachers were asked to complete the same scale as they might predict the child would answer each item. The correlation between teacher and child responses was fairly low ($r = .40$, not much better than chance), suggesting that teachers' perceptions about their students' social development and self-concept may not always be as accurate as hoped (Hartup, 1996).

"Back to Cases": Martin

In Chapter 1, our second case study involved a little boy named Martin, who was overlooked for party invitations and generally seemed to be the archetypal socially withdrawn child. How would his social competencies be described? Has he been teased? Has he learned the rules of social communication? Is he inherently painfully shy, so that a fear of being embarrassed only exacerbates the problem for him? Does his self-image as a user of a cochlear implant "amplify" differences between himself and his peers? As with Fatima, at this point, all we have are questions. Before we look at finding some answers, this chapter will conclude with a brief section on the emotional development of children with hearing loss—and it will be noted how this aspect is clearly woven into the psychological and social aspects as well.

Emotional Development

The primary concern about the emotional development of children with hearing loss is the abstract nature of emotions coupled with language deficits experienced by most children with hearing loss. This dynamic can result in a limited experience in self-expression and a delay in emotional awareness and emotional understanding. One study showed a very dramatic delay, with the affective understanding of deaf 17-year-olds being equivalent to hearing first graders (Kusche, Garfield, & Greenberg, 1983). Researchers have shown that children with hearing loss may be less accurate in identifying others' emotional states than children without hearing loss, and may have a poorer understanding of affective words. Since understanding affective vocabulary was positively related to personal adjustment (Greenberg & Kusche, 1993), these findings reinforce our understanding of the contributions of communication to self-understanding. For example, a child might be very distraught about something that happened at school, and appear negative and sullen, but when his mother asks him to explain, he might only be able to say "I'm upset!" He might lack the affective vocabulary needed him to express himself and understand his own emotional state. This self-awareness needs to be established before understanding and empathizing with others can occur.

Adolescence: Everything Seems Intensified

Most of the research reviewed so far has been focused on elementary school children. The teen years present additional challenges, and heightens the intensity of existing ones. Ginott (1969) described adolescence as a "period of curative madness, in which every teenager has to remake his personality. He has to free himself from childhood ties with parents, establish new identification with peers, and find his own identity" (p. 25). This "curative madness" requires the teen to deal with autonomy, peer group affiliation, identity formation, occupational preparation, and physiologic changes (Altman, 1996). Self-consciousness increases, as uncertainty and mood swings. Teens without hearing loss may feel besieged with emotions that they find hard to articulate, and the presence of hearing loss can exacerbate teens' struggles for self-awareness and self-expression.

As indicated above, peer relationships take paramount importance for teens, yet these relationships may be strained when hearing loss is involved. Mothers have reported that their teenage children seemed less emotionally bonded to their friends when hearing loss was a variable, and also rated these friendships as higher in aggression (Henggeler, Watson, & Whelan, 1990). Being with other teens with hearing loss may be more important than expected, when we consider how peer relationships help teens define themselves. Most of the 220 mainstreamed students in one study indicated that they preferred to spend most of their time with other students with hearing impairment, finding these relationships deeper and more satisfying (Stinson, Whitmore, & Kluwin, 1996).

The desire to conform to group expectations seems to peak in ninth grade (Kimmel & Weiner, 1995). For teens with hearing loss, this desire will probably include the desire to reject amplification for the sake of conformity. This desire may also represent a struggle to accept oneself as a person with a disability. The "hearing aid effect" is probably still in play, although there is some evidence that the magnitude of negative effect has lessened in the last 10 years (Haley & Hood, 1986; Stein, Gill, & Gans, 2000). Overall, however, it is well known that "during adolescence, being different is generally not valued" (Coyner, 1993, p. 19).

When considering emotional development, Sanders (1993) suggests adopting this perspective: "Perhaps the most helpful way to consider the emotional behaviors of hearing impaired children is to assume that they represent the child's best effort to deal with an abnormal experience" (p 374).

"Back to Cases": Curtis

Curtis was our third case study, the teen who "flew off the handle" when he thought he perceived an insult. Was his emotional reaction a reflection of his insecurity about being new in the school, or the level of competition of the team? Or is he delayed in his ability to manage ambiguity and stress? As with the other cases, we will explore these questions in depth in Chapters 3 and 4.

Chapter Summary

- A range of studies have described concerns in the psychological, social, and emotional development of children with hearing loss.

- Children who are deaf or hard of hearing may experience several or none of these difficulties. Each child will have a unique set of circumstances.
- The purpose of this chapter is to help professionals know what they should look for and be able to identify concerns before minor problems escalate into major ones.

Learning Activities

Clarification Activities

With a learning partner, describe your understanding of self-concept, the hearing aid effect, and the effect of hearing loss on a child's emotional and social development.

Describe your primary concerns about deaf and hard of hearing teens. How much different are these concerns compared to young people without hearing loss?

Modeling Activity

Wear a visible hearing aid (or two if available) for a full day or longer. Make note of your impressions of your self-image and the reactions of strangers.

Writing Activity

Write a few paragraphs describing your day with hearing aids, and reflect on any unexpected or undesirable aspects of the day. If you planned on rereading this assignment a year from now, what would you want to make sure you remembered?

Practice/Feedback

Identify in your mind a specific deaf or hard of hearing child that you know well, and fill in the blanks of these incomplete sentences as you believe this child would:

I am happy when_____

I am sad when _____

The thing I like most in the world is _____

The thing I would most like to change is _____
Because I cannot hear too well, _____

Describe to a learning partner the sensation of empathy as you attempt this exercise. Did it require effort or was it easy? Are you certain or doubtful that these answers accurately represent this child?

Suggested Readings in the Psychology of Deafness

Garrison, W. M. & Tesch, S. (1978). Self-concept and deafness: A review of research literature. *Volta Review, 80,* 457–66.

Marschark, M. (1993). *Psychological development of deaf children.* New York: Oxford University Press.

Moores, D. & Meadow-Orlans, P. (Eds.) (1990). *Educational and developmental aspects of deafness.* Washington, DC: Gallaudet University Press.

Paul, P. V. & Jackson, D. W. (1993). *Toward a psychology of deafness.* Boston: Allyn & Bacon.

Schum, R. (1991). Communication and social growth: A developmental model of social behavior in deaf children. *Ear and Hearing, 12*(5), 320–327.

Vernon, M., & Andrews, J. (1990). *The psychology of deafness: Understanding deaf and hard of hearing people.* New York: Longman.

CHAPTER

3

Basic Counseling Skills: "Opening the Door"

LEARNING OBJECTIVES

Readers of this chapter will be able to:

1. Identify three counseling theories and their applications to children with hearing impairment and their parents.
2. Describe two ways to "open the door" to a conversation about personal adjustment concerns.
3. Describe the goals and procedures of a set of "door-opening" instruments.

In the previous chapter, we reviewed highlights in current research describing significant concerns for the psychological and social well-being of children with hearing loss. It is quite possible that most of the children we serve are well-adjusted and thriving, and their families have established a steady foundation to their lives. However, if only one child causes us to be concerned, that should be reason enough to make ourselves available for support. This chapter will describe how to provide that support, by enhancing counseling repertoires with personal adjustment counseling skills and focused informational counseling skills.

Beginning the Counseling Process

In Chapter 1, several steps were provided to guide us as we attain non-professional counseling skills. These were:

☑ Help children "tell their story"
☐ Help them clarify their problem
☐ Help them challenge themselves to solve the problem
☐ Help them set a goal
☐ Help them develop an "action plan"
☐ Observe as they implement the plan
☐ Help them evaluate the plan

The first item in the list—helping children tell their story—indicates the focus of this chapter. Because it is the foundation of all counseling success, we will spend significant effort to learn this subtle art.

For the sake of argument, let us assume that most professionals start from the same point as David Luterman (1996) during training:

> ". . . Counseling was something one did after obtaining a careful case history and administering the diagnostic tests. Counseling was always information based and involved an explanation of the audiogram and recommendations for follow-through. I don't recall if the graduate students were given an injunction not to deal with the client's feelings, but we behaved as though we were. If a client displayed feelings (e.g., by crying), we were to refer the client to the clinical psychologist. The message I received in my training program was that client affect was the province of social workers and psychologists, and that counseling by audiologists and speech pathologists was to be information based." (p. 1)

Without question, children with hearing loss need and ask for information at times. However, we have come to see that children with hearing impairment also need more than information at certain times in their lives. Both informational counseling and personal adjustment support will be described here. Before we proceed, however, a review of some basic counseling approaches will be provided, as well as a discussion on how each approach might be applied by nonprofessional counselors to children with hearing loss.

Basic Counseling Approaches: An Overview

Crowe (1997b) provides a comprehensive description of the wide range of counseling approaches, beginning with a discussion of the ground-breaking work in psychoanalytic theory developed by Freud, Jung, and Adler. Although there have been many permutations over the years, it is generally agreed that nonprofessional counseling can be approached from three different perspectives: the *behavioral* approach, the *person-centered* approach, and the *cognitive-rational* or *cognitive-behavioral* approach. Long (1996) sees these three types of counseling approaches as different attempts to affect growth in one of three components of our personalities: behavior, feeling, and thinking.

- The behavioral approach (based on Skinner's principles of operant conditioning) seeks to change behaviors (actions and "doing").
- The humanist or person-centered approach (as developed by Carl Rogers) seeks to help in adjusting to affective experience (feelings, emotions, and existential "being").
- The cognitive approach (developed by Albert Ellis) seeks to change ways of thinking (thought processes, beliefs, and "choosing").

Following is a brief explanation of each approach, and a discussion of each as it might apply to nonprofessional counselors of children with hearing impairment.

Behavioral Approach

The principles of operant conditioning are familiar to the general population, and are routinely used in classrooms in the form of behavior modification. B. F. Skinner took Pavlov's principles of classical conditioning (training animals to react consistently to environmental stimuli) and developed a system of operant conditioning principles designed to shape human behavior (Skinner, 1938, 1953). By providing or withholding rewards or reinforcers, counselors have aimed to help individuals desist in maladaptive behaviors using token rewards to establish a pattern of preferred behaviors. As these behaviors become established, the token reward schedule is gradually reduced and the use of social reinforcers (social acceptance, social praise, self-esteem) is increased.

Applying the Behavioral Approach.   Behavior modification strategies are commonly used with children with hearing loss to establish desired behaviors such as increasing the use of hearing aids and developing responsibility for hearing aid care. These strategies have helped parents and teachers demonstrate concepts that are difficult to explain to a child with a limited vocabulary (such as consequences of one's behavior, controlling impulses, and so on).

The behavioral approach does not need to be limited to the management of undesired personal behaviors; it can also be used to promote prosocial behaviors as well. For instance, Martin (one of our case studies) is a child who appeared to be overlooked by other children, to all appearances more benignly neglected than actively rejected. His shyness or lack of confidence was adversely affecting potential friendship development. If we assume that this bothers him, and confirm from him directly that in fact it does, he might benefit from some support on developing behaviors that would be perceived as more friendly. Has he invited anyone to his house to play? Does he need practice approaching a group at a swing set? Is he doubtful that he would understand the rules of a kick-ball game and so avoids the game entirely? Does he retreat to the safety of a book in order to reduce the risk of embarrassment from misunderstandings in a group activity? We would need to know Martin's perspective, but a goal-and-reward system, and a safe environment in which to practice skills, might help him take small steps toward peers and peer activities, with long-lasting (possibly lifelong) effects (McGinnis & Goldstein, 1984). Examples could include (1) asking Martin to identify one person he would feel comfortable talking to at lunch, (2) decide on one prosocial behavior (ask to join the child and share a dessert), and (3) rewarding that effort with a sticker or other token. Martin then decides on the next small social risk, is rewarded for that effort again, and so on until the social successes are rewards unto themselves. This kind of support may have everything or nothing to do with the existence of a hearing loss; careful listening is needed to find out.

The next two approaches will consider applications with parents as well as with children; however, the behavioral approach is not to be applied to parents here, because it is not appropriate for a nonprofessional counselor to attempt to modify a parent's behaviors.

Person-Centered Approach

In the 1940s, Carl Rogers, strongly influenced by Maslow (particularly his principles of self-actualization) as well as his years of observation in the field, began to develop a different approach to counseling, one that positioned the client rather than the counselor as "expert." His approach assumed three clinician characteristics:

1. *Congruence.* Counselors are to be genuine in their clinical interactions, and must not maintain a professional distance or operate under false pretenses. They honestly convey their attitudes and opinions, giving the client every reason to trust them.

2. *Unconditional positive regard,* or "valuing the client" with no criticism for what one says or feels. The respect inferred in this condition includes the following behaviors:
   - Assume the client's goodwill
   - Refrain from judgment
   - Keep the client's agenda in focus (Egan, 1998)

   Unconditional positive regard does *not* mean one must fully agree with a child or parent, only that he or she is accepted, "warts and all."

   An example of positive unconditional regard was modeled by Rogers himself on a videotaped interview (American Association for Counseling and Development, 1982). He was conversing with an old friend, who asked at one point, "Let's try out your approach—I will start by telling you about my new job." He proceeded to explain that as a newly appointed president of a university, he found himself at odds with the expectation of his staff. They preferred him to keep a distance from the day-to-day concerns, but he preferred to be "in the trenches." He was feeling some pressure to be something he was not. He stopped his narrative for a moment and said, "I guess that must sound strange . . ." and Rogers responded, "It's not for me to say, it's how you are feeling right now." His colleague visibly relaxed upon hearing that verbal permission to say what he wanted, that no one was going to criticize him.

3. *Empathy.* Empathy is usually described as "putting oneself in another's place," or considering carefully how things are for someone else at this particular moment; that is, "the sincere attempt by clinicians to share in a client's inner feelings from within the client's internal frame of reference; clinicians experience both the inner feelings of clients and their own inner response to the client's feelings" (Crowe, 1997a, p.110).

Rogers (1961, 1986) reported that when these three conditions are in place—clinician congruence, unconditional positive regard, and empathy—client change can be affected. He held that each person has

the internal resources for health and growth, and the ability to identify and solve one's problems, if provided a supportive environment.
The role of the counselor then is to facilitate growth by providing the
conditions described above and create that safe nonjudgmental environment.

Applying the Person-Centered Approach.   The metaphor of a spotlight is a useful one to keep in mind when considering this approach
(Stone, Patton, & Heen, 1999). A spotlight can be shared by more than
one person, but when that happens, direct attention is dispersed rather
than focused on one individual. Recall Rogers' friend saying "I know
that must sound strange. . . ." Rogers actively stayed out of the spotlight by declining to express his opinion on the subject ("It's not for
me to say"), while intentionally keeping it focused on his friend ("It's
how you are feeling right now").

The person-centered approach would require us, then, to keep
the spotlight on the child or parent, and refrain from interjecting ourselves (our opinions, advice, recommendations, and so on) into that
light. For example, consider the following comment to Fatima:

"You need to cheer up and eat something."

This comment is intended to express concern, and the "spotlight" may seem to be focused on Fatima, but in reality the speaker
has inserted his or her advice, and now both the speaker and Fatima
are sharing the spotlight. In fact, the speaker is dominating it: "I know
what you should be doing about your life, you should listen to me."
As soon as we say, "You need to . . ." or "You should . . . ," we have
imposed our personality on another and have stopped attending to
what that person may want to say.

Compare that comment to this one: "You seem pretty blue lately"
(or "distracted" or "worried" or "as if something is bothering you").
Here, rather than jockeying for the spotlight, the speaker focuses only
on Fatima: an observation that something seems wrong, an expression of concern, and an implied offer to listen if she wants to talk (Figure 3.1).

These principles do not change when interacting with parents.
Congruence, unconditional positive regard, and empathy are conditions that can help many individuals tell their story. For instance, the
following example has the professional assert her "expert opinion" in

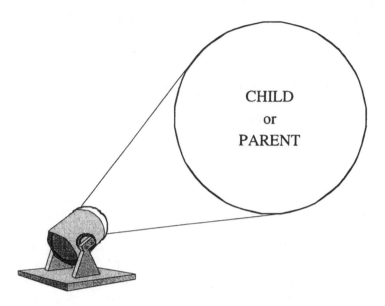

CHILD
or
PARENT

FIGURE 3.1   Keeping a spotlight on the child

response to a parent's comment, and no evidence of any of these conditions is apparent:

Scene: An Individualized Education Plan (IEP) meeting. A mother arrives, late and harried, for her appointment, and begins with this comment about her six year old daughter:

> MOTHER: Ashley hasn't been wearing her hearing aids for the last three weeks or so.
>
> PROFESSIONAL: She simply has to wear them every waking moment, and it's up to you to make sure that she does. She is probably in a little power struggle with you right now and you have to let her know who is boss.

This response does not assume the parent's goodwill or intentions to do "the right thing," but instead implies a judgment of incompetence. It does not focus on the parent's agenda, only on the professional's. If the mother attempts to answer this diatribe, she will likely be defensive and resentful for being chastised. She "opened a door" to her story, but the professional aggressively (and some might say arrogantly) slammed it shut, although, in her defense, it would appear that the professional is being congruent as a person who cared about Ashley's well-being.

Let's have the professional be congruent (true to self as a caring professional), *and* demonstrate unconditional positive regard:

> **MOTHER:**   Ashley hasn't been wearing her hearing aids for the last three weeks or so.
>
> **PROFESSIONAL:**   What's been going on lately?

What will the answer be? If we respect the complications of family life (empathy), it would be no surprise to hear any of the following:

- My father-in-law has been in the hospital and we have spent all our time there or with Ashley's grandmother. I'm just exhausted.
- We just got a new dog who not only is not house broken, but seems to want to slobber all over her hearing aids every time he gets close to Ashley. Would that ruin them? What should I do?
- Ashley had to get a couple teeth pulled and that seemed to be very painful, longer than the dentist led me to believe. She's just starting to eat without pain but for a time there, she was so cranky and sick-like. She didn't seem to have the energy to cope with her hearing aids.

What will be revealed will be the state of affairs with parent and child right now. Perhaps it is just a temporarily turbulent span of time that will run its course. Positive unconditional regard lets the parent know that the professional believes in her ability to reestablish stability. An empathic response to any of these explanations would indicate this: "You sound pretty overwhelmed right now. Is there anything I can do to help?"

Instead of a short-term disruption, perhaps mother and daughter really have reached an impasse: "It feels like Ashley and I are in a power struggle over the hearing aids right now, and everything I try just makes it worse. What can I do?" If she knew the professional was quick to judge her parenting abilities, she would not likely ask for advice. But because she feels unconditionally accepted, she seeks out this professional in a "learning-readiness" mind-set. A person-centered approach in counseling might result in invaluable opportunities to understand both parent and child concerns.

Rational Emotive Behavioral Therapy (REBT)

The rational emotive behavioral therapy (REBT) approach is based on the theory that a person's thoughts, feelings, and behaviors are interrelated. Developed in the 1950s (Ellis, 1962), this approach suggests that the way individuals think and feel about circumstances will affect their subsequent behaviors. Kelly (1992) provides this explanation: "When beliefs are expressed in absolute terms . . . or as inviolate rules of living . . . individuals may fail to see alternatives for responding to events. Cognitive counseling seeks to provide clients with alternative ways of thinking by teaching them to recognize and challenge their faulty beliefs and attitudes. . . . (p. 43–44)."

The REBT approach strives to help individuals examine unrealistic expectations, negative attitudes, and self-defeating assumptions, and learn how to see more options in a more positive frame of mind. Clients are prompted to use logic and reasoning to help move toward decision making and action by learning to attack irrational belief systems "head on."

The four most common types of irrational beliefs are these:

1. A person cannot imagine a situation being worse than it is already is. The situation or circumstance in question is virtually intolerable.
2. A person cannot imagine enduring a particular situation, much less being happy in this situation.
3. A person will likely be highly self-critical and critical of others, and ungenerous or unforgiving of mistakes.
4. A person will likely think only in absolutes (I must be right all the time, everything must be perfect, life must always go the way I had planned).

It doesn't take much imagination to see how these self-imposed limitations can negatively influence behaviors and overall satisfaction with life.

Some of the strategies used to help an individual see things from a more productive point of view are to challenge the assumptions expressed. For example:

CHILD: I can't wear that FM thing, kids will make fun of me.
ADULT: How do you know that?

Or:

> **CHILD:** There's no way I'm going to wear this cochlear implant anymore.
>
> **ADULT:** What is the worst thing that could happen if you did?

Clark (1994) describes how the practice of *saying* things differently can help a person *think about* things differently. The simple substitution of the word "and" for the word "but" allows the speaker to consider two conditions as allowably concurrent instead of mutually exclusive. For example:

> **CHILD:** I know those hearing aids help me but I hate the way they look.

This statement essentially rules out the consideration of hearing aid use: how they look overrides their benefits. What if we ask the child to rephrase that statement like this:

> **CHILD:** I know those hearing aids help me, and I hate the way they look.

This version gives full acknowledgment of a child's feelings, and also allows for the possibility that one can hate how the devices look *and still use them.* Before, the child had established a hard and fast position; now, the child can think more flexibly about enduring the "social costs" of using visible amplification devices.

Another helpful way to change language use is to replace words like *should, ought,* and *must,* with more flexible words such as *preference, desirable,* or *convenient.* Instead of insisting on the unrealistic expectation, "I must always be able to hear everything the teacher says," a child might be encouraged to say instead, "It would be convenient to be able to hear the teacher all the time—and most of the time I do." Or, if a teen may worry, "I should look like everyone else, and that means not wearing hearing aids," there might be less pressure to bear if the teen tried to see the situation more flexibly: "I would prefer to look like all the other kids, and I do, mostly."

People frequently reframe their situation with language to help them face a difficult situation:

- The doctor said my son will always have a hearing loss, but that's OK, at least it can be managed, it's not life-threatening like cancer.

- Our car was wrecked in a bad accident, we're just glad no one got hurt.

If the speaker in either situation did believe the circumstance was intolerable or unalterably devastating, he or she would be incapable of problem solving and finding ways to cope.

Combes and Gonzales (1994) describe three ways in which a person's perceptions can be modified. One of them was described above (helping a person see and describe longstanding or "old" experiences in new ways). The other two strategies are:

- *Changing the environment.* For example, in the school setting, the environment can actively express either acceptance and accommodation for a child with a hearing loss, or an attitude of inconvenience, resentment, and resistance. These environments usually are a reflection of the people in them, as well as how they choose to help or not help a child. A child's self-perception can be positively influenced by observing that her teacher insists that noise levels be controlled, that only one child will speak at a time, and that PA announcements are put in writing. She "gets the message" from this teacher that these listening conditions can be managed, and will be more likely to perceive that "If my teacher thinks hearing well is worth this trouble and effort, so will I."
- Conversely, a child's perception is negatively affected when people in her environment indicate that they would rather not "be bothered" by reasonable accommodations. A child's self-concept is undermined by teacher who sighs or rolls his or her eyes when reminded to use an FM microphone, for instance, or who, when asked to repeat instructions, does so in a sarcastic tone of voice. If at all possible, a change from a negative to a supportive, positive environment should be made if a child is having a difficult time.
- *Providing intervention from significant others.* In addition to the usual "significant others" in a child's life—family, friends and neighbors, religious leaders, teachers—intervention can also include support from (1) peers with hearing loss, (2) mentoring from older children/young adults with hearing loss (as in Big Brother/Big Sister programs), or (3) introductions to accomplished adults with hearing loss. Expanding the definition of "significant others" to include other persons with hearing loss gives us the opportunity to learn from those who have "been there." They can share their

own stories and perspectives, and describe alternative points of view, thereby giving children material to reflect on as a way to modify their own perspectives.

Scene: High school auditorium, "College Night." The audience consists of middle and high school deaf and hard of hearing students. Several guest speakers, all of whom have hearing impairment, have come to the podium, including one who says:

> SPEAKER: I always wanted to create things, but I wasn't really artistic. In my sophomore year in college, I took a computer class and learned a program that architects use to design buildings and remodelings. That's how I knew I wanted to do this for a living, so I changed majors and I will graduate with my degree next year.
>
> AUDIENCE: (thinks) If this person, who is only a little older than I am, is telling me that college is hard work but she knew her hearing loss was not going to keep her from her goal of being an architect. . . . maybe I can think that way about myself.

Applying REBT.   Let's return to our story about Curtis, the high school student who tried out for and the school track team. It could be said that his overreaction to a comment made by a teammate was based on an irrational thought: that the only thing this teammate could possibly have said had been an insult. When Curtis realized his mistake, he experienced another irrational thought: the only way to address this misunderstanding was to drop the team altogether.

If he explained the situation, a "tuned in" listener could help him reconsider his "absolute" thinking and show how this was controlling his decisions. This approach might be more effective with an adult who actually witnessed the misunderstanding, or had rapport with Curtis about things unrelated to track. In other words, Curtis would not likely tell the track coach, "I've decided to drop out of track because I misunderstood a teammate and now am too embarrassed to be around him." However, another adult or a friend—one of the "significant others" mentioned earlier—could help him talk it out and see things differently.

On occasion, parents may also benefit from an REBT approach when it is observed that irrational or absolute thinking is adversely affecting their adjustment and acceptance. Parents may express perceptions such as:

- I could never learn sign language, it looks too hard.
- If I home-school my child, I can protect him from being teased by other kids.
- I can never forgive myself, I know I caused this hearing loss because I drank some wine at a wedding while I was pregnant.

Parents bear unknown sorrow, and some days it is easier to handle than others. In some frames of mind, a direct attempt to help them "think about it differently" could be perceived as an attack or a challenge, as in:

> **PARENT:**   I could never learn sign language, it looks too hard.
>
> **PROFESSIONAL:**   What could be the worse thing that could happen if you tried to learn? Or, How do you know for sure?

If not worded with care, the professional's comment could sound like criticism. The REBT approach is not as complicated when used with the child with hearing loss, but a parent brings a wide range of additional emotional concerns (guilt, confusion, grief, vulnerability, and so on), and the professional will want to think about this approach carefully before using it.

Which Approach to Use?

We have reviewed three very different counseling approaches, and the reader may be familiar with others as well. At this point, one may ask, "Which approach is right? Which approach should I learn? How will I know which approach to use?" Following Luterman's (1996) advice may be more helpful than worrying about technique per se:

> The key to counseling is the congruence of the counselor. As I become more congruent, technique slips away, or, more accurately, becomes incorporated into everything I do. . . . The importance of the congruent professional far exceeds the value of any diagnostic test or specific techniques in counseling. If the literature on the desirable personality characteristics of the counselor were examined, it would appear that no one would qualify unless one could also qualify for sainthood. . . . One [only] needs to be a caring individual who does not impose beliefs on others, who maintains a constant awareness of self, and who does not hide behind the artificiality of being a professional. (p. 178)

In other words, as Rogers has been quoted, "The most effective technique which leads to insight on the part of the client is the one which demands the utmost in self-restraint on the counselor's part." This can be interpreted to mean: the less the counselor talks and tries to solve a person's problems, the more the person can talk and hear oneself talk, and the more likely he or she will achieve self-understanding and develop one's own answers.

The approach espoused in this book would best be described as individualistic; that is, any approach which feels comfortable to the professional and which promotes conversation with a child while actively, reflectively listening. Each adult will be different, each child will be different, and each concern will be different. It will be up to the professional to find the right match for the circumstance at hand.

But, while we won't overstress technique per se, as we compare and contrast these approaches, we should ask ourselves: In each approach, who is in control? Who is assumed to know best? When applied to hearing loss, who is in control and who knows best? Ultimately, who owns this hearing loss, the child, the parent, the professional? Since our long-term goal is to facilitate the transition of a parent's ownership of the hearing loss to the child as the child grows, we will want to select counseling approaches that advance that goal.

"Let's Think About Doors"

In Chapter 1, the first step in the counseling process was identified as helping a child "tell his or her story." To help us consider *how* to help a child tell his or her story, a "door" metaphor will be used. The remaining part of this chapter will describe strategies designed to "open a door" to a conversation—that is, help children "tell their story." Strategies designed to "keep the door (conversation) open" will be presented in Chapter 4.

As mentioned in Chapter 1, nonprofessional counseling has two goals: to convey information and also to provide personal adjustment support. Careful listening is required to know which is needed at a given moment. In counseling, this kind of activity is called "listening with the third ear"—a particularly meaningful concept for those working with children with hearing impairment (Reik, 1949)!

Informational counseling will be discussed later, because it is the easier activity of the two, and because personal adjustment concerns

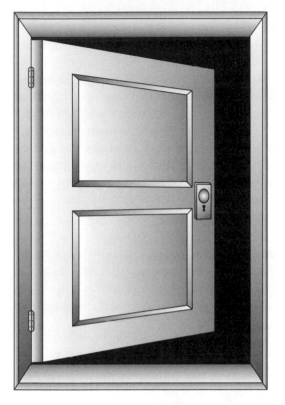

FIGURE 3.2   Opening doors

must be addressed before children can focus on the information directed toward them. Children are not likely to learn new information if they are upset and if their feelings have not been acknowledged (Faber & Mazlish, 1995). And those feelings are not "just some noisy byproduct" of a situation (Stone et al., 1999); rather, at this moment, feelings *are* the situation, and if they are not acknowledged first, little progress will be made in learning or problem solving.

"Opening the door" to a child's story can occur two ways:

1. We can "hear a knock" by attending carefully to expressions of personal adjustment concerns.
2. We can extend an invitation by actively evoking conversation about these concerns.

Both approaches will be described below. Before we go further, how-ever, we have to think about what happens to *us* when we "open the door" to a counseling conversation. Are we ready and willing to re-ceive the expressions of potentially upsetting or confusing emotions? We must use our own emotional strength to serve as nonprofessional counselors. Once a child entrusts us with an expression of his or her feelings, we cannot turn our back. We want to be fully aware that some days, because of our own pressures, worries, and stressors, we do not have this emotional strength for others, and that we need to maintain realistic expectations of our abilities to help.

"Hearing a Knock"

For our purposes, "hearing a knock" (as in "tuning in") means perceiv-ing the affect as well as the content of a statement. Even the most ca-sual observer will notice that much of what children say discloses their affective state. It is relatively easy to "hear" the emotion conveyed in the following examples:

> "This is my favorite TV show."
> "Not oatmeal again! We have it every morning, practically."
> "No way I'm wearing that shirt to school."
> "I swam five laps for the first time today."

Note that these words were not actually spoken, yet we still "heard" them:

> I am **enthusiastic** about this TV show.
> I am **unhappy** about the breakfast menu.
> I am **upset** about wearing that shirt.
> I am **proud** of myself for finishing those five laps.

These emotions were not stated aloud, but we could still perceive them. Yet sometimes emotions are not as apparent. For example, what emo-tions might underlie these statements?

> "My father stops signing to me when we go to McDonald's."
> "Do I have to wear these hearing aids all day?"
> "I've never been invited to a birthday party."

If we are tuning in, we can perceive that there is more here than the words indicate: that is, the emotions behind the words are as important, if not more so, than the literal meaning of the words themselves. The phrase, **if we are tuning in**, needs to be stressed, because we need to be aware that this kind of listening does not come naturally or easily to most of us. In the next chapter, we will examine why this kind of careful listening is hard to do.

As a point of contrast, compare the previous statements with these:

"Can you show me how to change the tire on my bicycle?"
"Have you seen my soccer shoes?"
"When did the teacher say our book report was due?"

These seem like fairly straightforward requests for information, although it would not be surprising if they were expressed with a range of emotions as well. Children are not expected to be reserved or dispassionate about the circumstances around them.

Parents may also approach professionals with "door-opening" comments, and the same analysis would be conducted—that is, asking oneself if they are only requests for information, or is there affect involved as well? Sometimes it can be hard to tell; on the surface, this statement could just be a request for information:

"Will Maya have to do this auditory training stuff the rest of her life?"

This parent may really just want to know the answer to this question: do adults obtain auditory training as well as children? Am I expected to know when she is "done"? If so, how will I know? However, there may also be a level of frustration, worry, or despair— maybe the real question, unspoken, is, "Will Maya struggle with a hearing loss for the rest of her life?"

Some comments and questions are not as complicated. Again, as a point of contrast, straightforward requests for information that are heard all the time include these examples:

- How long should we expect batteries to last?
- Does the new principal know anything about hearing loss and learning?
- Have you heard about a vaccine for ear infections?

And some comments or questions are obviously highly affective:

- When I was told Amelia had a hearing loss, well, it was like dragging dead fish through pond scum.
- Charlie's grandmother cries every time she sees those hearing aids on him. She can't seem to get over it, and that upsets everyone else.
- There are days when I really understand that old saying, "Life is a roller coaster and sometimes I just want to get off."

In all of these examples, parents and children are opening the door to a conversation with the professional. When a professional has tuned into the nature of the comment or question, conducting an on-the-spot analysis, he or she is using a skill called **differentiation**. In counseling, all success depends on the careful differentiation of the opening remarks: if we don't perceive the nature of the comment, we cannot expect to respond to it appropriately.

"Hearing a knock," then, is the habit or conscious effort of evaluating the nature of a comment: when a child or parent initiates a communication, is he or she asking for information only, or is a personal adjustment concern embedded within? Our response should be dependent on what we hear, and in the next chapter we will discuss our responses. But right now, what can one do when a child appears to be having some difficulties, but is not especially forthcoming about what these difficulties might be? In other words, although we are becoming concerned about what we see, the child is not "opening the door" on his own. The next step in nonprofessional counselor can be to seek ways to help a child "tell his story," by evoking or eliciting some conversation or reactions from the child, or "actively opening the door."

Actively Opening the Door

To help find out how a child is doing, professional counselors have a range of materials to use, such as the *Piers-Harris Children's Self-Concept Scale* (Piers, 1984), which uses an 80-item questionnaire format to assess how children feel about themselves with respect to physical appearance, intelligence, school status, anxiety, popularity, happiness, and so on. It is a standard instrument among school psychologists and counselors for children ages 8–18, with and without hearing impairment.

The "Self-Description Questionnaire II (SDQ-II)" (Marsh, 1992) looks at several dimensions of self-concept as well, including physical ability and appearance, same-sex and opposite-sex relationships, parental relations, emotional stability, and honesty/trustworthiness. It is designed for preteens, ages 7–12; no data are available on using this questionnaire with children who are deaf or hard of hearing.

Nonprofessional counselors have a few materials available to them as well. For example, the *Meadow-Kendall Social-Emotional Assessment Inventories for Deaf and Hearing Impaired Students* (Meadow-Orlans, 1983) carefully describes child behaviors and personality traits that might support or substantiate overall concerns for a child's development. This instrument asks teachers to answer as true or false 59 statements such as "[child] relates well to peers and is accepted by them," or "[child] has generally acceptable emotional ranges." The *Meadow-Kendall* was normed on over 1,800 deaf children, and is the only instrument specifically designed to rate the social and emotional development of deaf children in comparison to other deaf children.

The *Social Skills Rating System* (Gresham & Elliot, 1990) includes not only teacher reports but also solicits input from parents and the students themselves. The scales consider social skills (such as cooperation, assertiveness, responsibility, empathy, and self-control), problem behaviors (such as aggression, anxiety, and hyperactivity), and academic competence. The self-report section gives a student the opportunity to describe social skills on the basis of frequency (how often: never, sometime, very often) and importance (not important, important, critical).

Certainly teacher reports are invaluable in obtaining a description of behaviors and concerns. However, to go beyond these data, to help a child "tell his or her story" in order to understand the child's perspective, as well as help develop self-awareness and skills in self-expression, we need to consider ways to actively open the door to a conversation with that child. There is a real challenge in opening a conversation with a child when the concern is personal or emotional or upsetting. Even when the content is not personal or emotional, as with the classic example, "What did you do in school today?" (the usual answer being "Nothing"), opening a conversation can be difficult. How effective then will these openers be?

- Why are you in such a bad mood?
- Is something wrong?
- Are you OK? You looked like you swallowed a lemon.

Most likely, a child will dodge these kinds of questions with a noncommittal response, because he or she did not perceive a nonjudgmental listener. Direct questions can easily put children on the defensive, or make them feel uncomfortable enough to avoid the situation.

This concept may be familiar to those who have studied research on the interactions between mothers and infants with hearing loss. Without intervention, mothers have been found to overcontrol the topic of conversation, as well as overcontrol responses and turn taking. Mothers' responses are frequently unrelated to the child's previous response, and their comments are unrelated to what the child is looking at. The most effective interventions were those which taught the mother to adapt her response to the action and eye gaze of the child (Jamieson, 1995). This principle is being adapted herein: to make our behaviors and responses contingent on the child's behaviors and responses.

Three "tell me your story" approaches are described in the following section, and are offered as a way of exploring the topics of:

- Friendship development
- Self-awareness and personal concerns
- Readiness for change

It is essential to remember that none of these strategies are tests! If we think of them as door-openers, we will be more likely to elicit conversation from children.

"Door Openers"

Talking About Friendships: *Children's Peer Relationship (CPR) Scale*

Rationale.   The *Children's Peer Relationship Scale (CPR Scale)* was developed to provide a mechanism that might "open the door" to a conversation with a child about friendship development (English, 2001). As we learned in Chapter 2, children with hearing impairment tend to perceive themselves as less likeable, having less social status, and having fewer friends than their peers without hearing impairment. The *CPR Scale* was developed to provide a means to broach the sensitive topics of self-concept and friendship development, by offering an opportunity for children to describe their concerns in a nonthreatening, nonjudgmental environment. The items are loosely adapted from a socioemotional adjustment scale developed by Sanders (1993).

As mentioned earlier, it is essential to emphasize that the *CPR Scale* is not a test. Rather, it is a set of discussion points designed to help children consider and identify their perceptions, and express them to a trusted adult. When administrating the *CPR Scale*, rapport, trust, and positive regard must exist between the administrator and child.

The *CPR Scale* has eight discussion points with the choice of three responses, designed to reflect a positive, neutral, or negative perception. The complete version of the CPR can be found the Appendix, and a summary or report form will be found in Figure 3.3.

The first item ("I like school/School is OK/I don't like school") is a warm-up topic, and responses may or may not have much to do with peer relationships or self-concept per se. Administrators are encouraged to elicit at least one comment about each discussion point, to give the child an opportunity to expand upon the response given. Obviously, the more conversation on a particular point, the more opportunity for self-expression—in other words, not only "open the door" to their story but also "keep the door open" as much as possible.

It has been noted that when face-to-face conversation is difficult, it can help for two people to direct their mutual attention on a neutral "third thing," something that both parties can think and talk about. This approach reduces the anxiety often felt when disclosing personal information. The *CPR Scale* was designed with this phenomenon in mind.

Administration.   The *CPR Scale* should be administered in a quiet room with no distractions, **sitting side-by-side** (not face-to-face) with the child at a table. Provide a marker or pencil for the child, and give these instructions:

> I was wondering how you would answer these questions. I will read them aloud to you (or ask readers to do this aloud on their own), and then I would like you to checkmark the box that describes you best. We can take our time and talk about your check marks for as long as you want to.

FIGURE 3.3 *Children's Peer Relationship (CPR) Scale*

CPR Scale*
"Children's Peer Relations Scale"
Record Form

Responses collected by: _____   Date _____

Child: _____   Age _____

Circle child's responses to these items:

1.   I like school.
       School's OK.
       I don't like school.

2.   I have some good friends in school.
       I have one good friend in school.
       I don't have good friends in school.

3.   I have a best friend.
       I sort of have a best friend.
       No one is really my best friend.

4.   Mostly, other children like me.
       Sometimes, other kids don't like me.
       Other children don't really like me.

5.   I usually play with friends after school.
       Sometimes I play with friends after school.
       I don't see anyone after school.

6.   Other kids don't tease me about my hearing loss.
       Sometimes, other kids tease me about my hearing loss.
       Other kids tease me a lot about my hearing loss.

7.   I know other kids who have hearing loss.
       I know one other kid who has a hearing loss.
       I don't know any other kids who have hearing loss.

8/ha. I really like wearing my hearing aids.
       My hearing aids are OK.
       I hate having to wear hearing aids.

8/ci. I really like wearing my cochlear implant.
       My cochlear implant is OK.
       I hate having to wear a cochlear implant.

Adapted from Sanders, D. A. (1993). Socioemotional adjustment guide (p. 376). *Management of hearing handicap: Infants to elderly* (3rd ed.). Englewood Cliffs, NJ: Prentice Hall.

To reiterate: Be sure the child understands that this is not a test, and that no answer is right or wrong. Provide opportunity for the child to describe or identify any concerns by eliciting a remark or comment about each item. Use neutral prompts such as "Really? How so?," "That's a problem?" or "I didn't know that, can you tell me about that?" Avoid asking "Why?" since that could make a child defensive, and avoid discounting their responses: for instance, if a child indicates he or she doesn't have any friends, a response such as "That's not true, you are always being invited to birthday parties," does not respect his or her perception. As Stone et al. (1999) put it, this kind of conversation is not about getting the facts straight, but how the child perceives the facts: it is "not about what is true, but what is important" (p. 10).

After the child has left, transfer his or her responses to the Record Form, and add any comments as well. The forms with the child's check marks can then be destroyed if considered appropriate.

Advantages.   Field testing of the *CPR Scale* suggested that it is a non-threatening way to "open a door" to a conversation on friendship development (English, 2001). As long as they had an existing warm rapport with the child, adults were able to elicit a great deal of conversation about friendships. Interestingly, when teachers were asked to predict how a child might respond to each item, their answers were not in high agreement with the child's actual answers ($r = .40$, only slightly better than chance). Therefore, the *CPR Scale* could reveal concerns that teachers may not be aware of.

Disadvantages.   The *CPR Scale* addresses only friendship development and (minimally) self-image, and does not directly promote exploration of other psychosocial concerns. Not just any adult can successfully administer this tool, since rapport must exist beforehand. In addition, field testers reported the caution that the administrator must be alert to a tendency of discounting a child's perceptions. If a child indicates that he or she has few friends, we cannot argue this response in an attempt to make the child "feel better." For example, if a child reports having few friends, the adult does not help by reminding, "You see all those kids in the scouting group, those are friends, aren't they?" (The "pitfalls" of inappropriate reassurance will be discussed in Chapter 4.) The adult has to be ready for the possibility that the answers might not be upbeat, and that the child may disclose insecurity, loneliness, or lack of awareness of what social skills are requisite for making and keeping friends. In addition, what might be disclosed could be a temporary falling-out of a normally stable friendship—another reason why the adult needs to know the child well.

Talking About Self-Awareness and Personal Concerns: *"I Start/You Finish"*

Rationale.   In Chapter 2, Loeb and Sarigiani (1986) provided evidence indicating that children with hearing loss had lower self-esteem and perceived themselves as less likeable than children without hearing loss. It appeared that communication difficulties set the stage for social isolation.

One of their measures was designed specifically for this study, but it was not given a name, so for simplicity's sake it will be identified here as the *I Start/You Finish* activity. This format is frequently used to encourage self-expression; for example, professional counselors have used versions of the *Rotter Incomplete Sentences Blank* (2d ed.)(1992) as an interview technique since the 1950s. Persons are asked to complete sentence stems such as, "If only I could. . . ." Or "I can usually. . . ." and the evaluator looks for patterns of stress or personal outlook. For our purposes, the *I Start/You Finish* activity can be an effective way of opening the door to a child's self-perception and self-awareness, and to facilitate the telling of his or her story.

Administration.   As with the *CPR Scale*, the *I Start/You Finish* activity should be administered in a quiet room with no distractions. Seating arrangements can be side-by-side, or at right angles in chairs, with or without a table. Sitting face-to-face on either side of a table or desk is not recommended. These instructions should be given:

> I have some sentences here that have no endings. I was wondering how you would complete them. I'll start them off and ask you to finish them for me. You can add more sentences to each one if you want; we can take our time and talk about your sentences for as long as you want. I will write down what you say to help me remember everything.

Again, as with the *CPR Scale*, make sure the child understands that this is not a test, and that no answer is right or wrong. Provide opportunity to the child to describe or identify any concerns by eliciting a remark or comment about each item. The open-ended sentences are provided in Figure 3.4.

FIGURE 3.4 *"I Start/You Finish"*

- I am happy when _____.

- I am sad when _____.

- The thing I like most in the world is _____.

- The thing I would most like to change is _____.

- Because I have a hearing problem _____.

Advantages.   The *I Start/You Finish* activity has the obvious advantage of open-endedness: that is, the child is not being directed to focus on any specific situation or concern, and is given permission to explore anything he or she chooses. If a child feels secure in the situation, he or she is likely to provide genuine answers, giving the adult an invaluable glimpse into the child's world, a better understanding of "this is what it is like to be me right now."

Disadvantages.   By the same token, the lack of direction or boundaries may make either the child or the adult feel uncomfortable. Adults should not attempt this kind of conversation-opener unless they are able to tolerate unpredictable outcomes and ambiguity. And if they perceive discomfort on the child's part, of course the activity quickly comes to a close.

Providing appropriate follow-up discourse will be discussed in the next chapter ("Keeping the Door Open").

Talking About Change: Using a "Readiness Scale"

Rationale.   The *Readiness Scale* can be used when a child is facing a change of any kind, or to bring a child into a decision-making process. These changes and decisions happen on a regular basis, although frequently they are imposed on children without their input. For example:

- "Fatima, you would hear your teacher better if you used an FM system. I've ordered one already, and it will probably arrive tomorrow."

■ "Martin, your teacher wants you go to math class with some older kids, isn't that great?"

If we place ourselves in these children's positions, we can easily imagine feeling unprepared for these events, to say nothing of feeling worried or resentful: "This may seem like a good idea to you, but no one asked me about it!" An instrument such as the *Readiness Scale* could help navigate some of these changes, and allow a certain amount of input from the child.

Administration.   As with the first two instruments, the *Readiness Scale* should be used in a confidential setting where the child has the adult's undivided attention. It is simply a scale from one to ten, as depicted in Figure 3.5, "1" representing complete rejection of a change or plan, and "10" representing 100 percent commitment and readiness. It can be presented in conjunction with the proposed change, with a question about how a child would rate him- or herself as being ready for it. A revisit of the above examples would go something like this:

■ "Fatima, I notice you are missing a lot of your teacher's instruction, and I would suggest that you try out an FM system. I have a system in my office and can get it ready for you tomorrow, but I want to know how you feel about it. If you used this arrow, ranging from 1–10, how ready would you be to try it out?"
■ "Martin, your teacher wants you go to math class with some older kids. That would be a pretty big change for you. On this scale of 1–10, how ready would you be to try this idea out?"

If a child's response falls anywhere from 1 to 7, we have a clear indication that some discussion needs to be developed before the

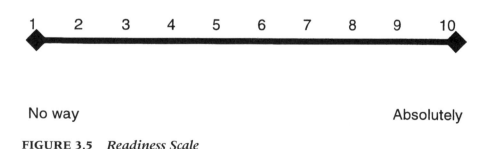

FIGURE 3.5   *Readiness Scale*

change is made. The rating provided by the child almost always includes an expression of his or her concerns about the situation, giving the adult more to work with:

- "Maybe a 4, I really don't like this idea much."
- "I suppose a 7, it sounds OK to me, basically."

Advantages.   Using a readiness scale gives a child the opportunity to understand herself or himself, and express that understanding. It can give the adult and child a focus, and an opportunity to practice problem solving and develop strategies to reach the "readiness goal." What will it take to help Fatima be ready to use an FM at least in some situations, part time or selectively? Obtain her active evaluation of its "social costs" versus "academic benefits"? What are *her* suggestions to move into this change? What steps could be taken to help Martin take a more challenging math class? Using a readiness scale as a starting point also promotes accountability: "When I first mentioned this, you said you were '8–9' ready, but it looks like you are having problems—do you have a different opinion now that we actually started? What do I need to know?"

Disadvantages.   The "1–10" concept is too abstract for younger children, and probably should not be used with children under the age of 8. Also, there is the risk that a child might indicate that under no circumstance will he or she ever be ready for this change, resulting in an apparent stalemate. If that is the child's expressed position, at least we know when we find ourselves struggling with passive-aggressive behaviors (e.g., forgetting homework) or sabotage (e.g., consistently "losing" the teacher's microphone).

Counseling with Information: Not to be Overlooked

The careful listener will know that not every issue for a child is an emotional one; sometimes they are only in need of information about their hearing loss or the development of communication strategies. Following are two instruments designed to "open the door" to a conversation about a variety of listening situations and possible solutions.

Like the instruments described above, these are not tests, but rather a set of prompts or discussion items.

Hearing Performance Inventory for Children (HPIC)

The *HPIC* (Giolas, Maxon, & Kessler, 1997) is a set of 31 pictures depicting a wide range of school listening situations. It was designed for children between the ages of 8–14, and because children are shown pictures, results are not adversely affected by reading limitations.

Administration.   The *HPIC* is administered by showing a set of pictures, one at a time, with these instructions:

> "I will be showing some pictures to you. I want you to look at the pictures and tell me if what you see ever happens in your class. If it does, I want you to tell me if it is always, a lot, sometimes, a little, or never hard for you to hear when that happens (p. 7)."

The first picture depicts a teacher at the front of a classroom pointing to words on a blackboard. Children are at their desks. The questions posed for this scenario are: "This teacher is talking in front of the class. Does your teacher do that? Is it hard to hear him speaking?"

Additional scenes depict a teacher giving directions for a test, writing on the blackboard and talking at the same time, and reading to the class. Other concerns are considered: Is it hard to hear another student give an answer in class? Can you hear the fire bell? Can you hear a movie shown in class, or hear in P.E. class, or in the hall or cafeteria? How hard is it to hear when your hearing aid is broken?

The child assigns a value from 1 to 5 in terms of difficulty to each scenario. Once the inventory is administered, the adult reviews situations identified as difficult. He or she will want to address the consequences of not hearing in these situations, the child's responses to the situations, and options to explore for communication repair strategies. Intervention supports the development of self-advocacy skills: if unable to understand the teacher, the child may need to work on how to let the teacher know about the problem. Teachers also get feedback from students' responses and are encouraged to consider their instructional methods in light of the difficulties noted.

The *HPIC* uses a set of well-drawn pictures to provide an opportunity for children to consider school situations from several perspectives, and provides much-needed practice in describing their problems and developing a problem-solving mindset. Its introduction lays out a few suggestions to begin rehabilitation and discussion. Pictures can be selected to represent school situations for children in elementary, middle, or high school levels. As a counseling tool, the administrator would need skills in reacting to the child's response, since it will not be constrained by a scale of answers.

With 31 pictures to discuss, the HPIC can seem too long for many children. Some of the scenes may not represent school life these days, so some of its pictures may appear dated.

Listening Inventories for Education (LIFE)

The *LIFE* (Anderson & Smaldino, 1998) was designed to expand upon the strengths of the *HPIC* (giving children the opportunity to self-report on a variety of listening conditions) by adding a teacher version, and by narrowing the focus of listening conditions to those most commonly found in school settings today. The student self-report helps identify listening challenges, and can be compared to the teacher report; a third inventory is a Teacher Opinion and Observation List, which helps document teachers' perceptions of the effects of interventions taken to improve listening conditions. The *LIFE* is primarily intended for elementary school age children.

Administration.   Like the *HPIC*, the *LIFE* presents a set of pictures (15 total), and the child's responses are obtained using a five point scale. Unlike the *HPIC*, however, the *LIFE* provides an alternative response method with the use of five different cartoon faces depicting "always easy" to "always difficult" (see Figure 3.6).

Following is a sample item to discuss and rate:

> The teacher is talking, but has his back to you. You cannot see the teacher's face. Tell me how well you can hear the words the teacher is saying.

The *LIFE* is relatively quick to administer (15 minutes), and can be used as an efficacy measure by obtaining student and teacher input

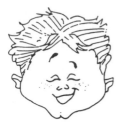
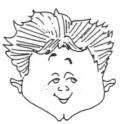
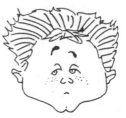

always easy   mostly easy   sometimes difficult

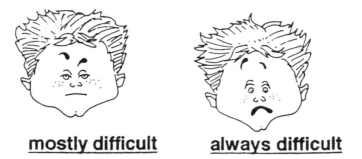

mostly difficult   always difficult

FIGURE 3.6   Five answers to items in the *Listening Inventories for Education (LIFE)*, Anderson & Smaldino (1998), reprinted by permission

before and after intervention measures (such as using a personal FM system or a trial period of classroom amplification). The teacher completes an "appraisal of listening difficulty" to consider attention span, classroom involvement, and so on. As with any closed-set instrument, topics may be constrained to those presented on cards.

Both inventories described above give children with hearing loss an important opportunity to consider their circumstances and discuss what they understand about them. While the focus of this book has been on personal adjustment counseling, it is not meant to diminish the value of content or informational counseling at any time, and professionals are exhorted to ensure that children do have the information they need to solve their hearing challenges.

"Door Openers" for Parents

Because hearing impairment usually is a new experience in their lives, parents are in the difficult position of "not knowing what they don't know." Parents frequently undergo what Atkins (1994) calls a "restructuring process" (p. 117)—adjusting to what the hearing impairment means to the family at this time. Their child's needs will change every month and every year, and parents report often feeling inadequate and ill-prepared for the challenges (Luterman, 1995). As the child grows, so do parental concerns: the child's social circle will widen, the need for "life skills" will increase, and differences between their child and children without hearing loss will become more and more apparent. Parents may be concerned about their child's self-image and self-concept as well as meeting the needs of other children in the family and managing work responsibilities and marital relationships.

To help parents collect and organize audiological information about their children, Flexer (1999) has developed a form for audiologists to complete for parent's records (pp. 98–102). The form asks for the types of tests that have been conducted to date, the kinds of stimuli used and the observations and results, estimations of pure tone averages, responses to Ling speech sounds, hearing aid data, and recommendations for listening activities. This systematic method of record keeping helps both parent and professional ensure that all information is shared and understood. This kind of form serves as an effective "door opener" to parental concerns, by providing basic information while considering questions about the future.

As fundamental information about hearing is obtained and absorbed (a parent's version of "Audiology 101"), the professional will want to keep the "information stream" primed, but also individualized as parents identify what is important to them at the moment. An effective "door opening" strategy is to develop a wide-ranging list or menu of relevant topics (including blank space to add other topics) offered for parental review, and disseminated with this request: "Do you want more information on this topic or other topics? If so, would you prefer (please check all that apply): a group presentation, a guest speaker, a set of written materials, a short pamphlet, a referral to an experienced parent, other?" This process will help parents obtain the information needed when that information is wanted.

The following is a very short list of topics parents might be interested in:

- For parents whose children are in grades K–2, topics might be include otitis media, communication skills, hearing aid problems,

FM systems, friendship development, and the special education/ IEP process.

- As children reach grades 3–6, the issues may grow to include reading and other academic concerns, involvement in sports, use of the telephone, and obtaining/using captioned television.
- Children in middle school and high school grades will also be contending with peer pressure concerns, self-identity, an increasing degree of independence and responsibility, career exploration, dating, and development of post-high school plans.

This menu-driven approach exemplifies the idea of *empowerment*, a concept that unfortunately has lost its impact from overuse but one that still resonates. By developing an informational program that parents can "tap into" as needed, professionals demonstrate their respect for parental choice and readiness to learn as new concerns present themselves. The opposite approach, professionals deciding what parents need to know, only distances both parties from the mutual goal of child success. Luterman (1996) puts it this way: "When the professional calls the shots, the parents become spectators" (p. 51).

Once the professional learns what parents want to learn, and how they want to learn it, he or she can draw on a wide range of materials. Four resources are described at the end of this chapter.

Finally, it would be remiss not to mention that a professional will want to have a referral system readily available if parents begin to demonstrate psychoemotional problems that exceed one's professional boundaries (Stone & Olswang, 1989) and require intervention by professional counselors.

Chapter Summary

- Three counseling approaches were reviewed: behavioral, person-centered, and cognitive (REBT), and each approach was considered as a way to help children with hearing loss.
- It is incumbent upon the professional to "hear a knock" or "tune in" and analyze a comment (differentiation) as either a request for information or an expression of a personal adjustment concern.
- To help a child tell his or her story as the beginning of the counseling process, three "door opening" strategies were presented.

- "Door openers" for parents by way of information-sharing will help keep the "information stream" primed and also provide opportunities to discuss concerns.

Learning Activities

Clarification Activity

Examples of different counseling approaches were applied to our case studies (Fatima, Martin, and Curtis) throughout this chapter, and are filled into spaces in the table below. Fill in the blanks to experiment with applications of these approaches with other children. Do some approaches seem to be a better match than others? Why or why not?

	Behavioral	Person Centered	REBT
Fatima		"You seem kinda blue."	
Martin	provide rewards for efforts in initiating play		
Curtis			Another way to handle situation?

Modeling Activity

Consult with someone you consider to be a good listener, and ask him or her to describe what is heard, in addition to "the facts," in the statements below.

- *Mr. Bonito, parent:* "For the first time in her short life, Lonnie was scoring at the top of a scale instead of the bottom on some therapy goals. Things seemed to be looking up, and then we heard our insurance claim was denied. We owe over $1,000 now."
- *Mrs. Clemson, parent:* "I love Michael, of course, but if I had known sooner that he was deaf, I wouldn't have had a second child—she's deaf too."
- *Sarah, age 12:* "No one else in school wears hearing aids."

- *Sam, age 16:* "I was thinking about applying for a job at the stadium, but what if no one there understands me when I talk to them?"
- *Mrs. Yamana, parent:* "If we agree to send our son to that special school, it would mean he'd spend more than 2 hours a day on the bus."
- *Mr. and Mrs. Best:* "The more sign language we learn, the more we realize how little we really know. How are we going to talk with our child when the topic is really serious or complicated?"

Writing Activity

What affective statements have you heard with your "third ear" when interacting with children or parents? Write down three statements that seem at least partly affective:

1. _____

2. _____

3. _____

Practice/Feedback

Read your three statements from the Writing Activity to a learning partner and obtain feedback: do these statements seem affective to your partner as well? What kinds of feelings or emotions does your partner hear, and are they same or different from what you heard? If different, what might account for that?

Four Informational Resources for Parents (see Reference Section for publishing information)

1. *Developmental Index of Audition and Listening (DIAL)* (Palmer & Mormer, 1998). The *DIAL* provides a description of typical auditory behaviors seen in different age groups (e.g., early-school-age children use the telephone meaningfully; late elementary-school-age children re-

spond to sirens for street safety and attend to the rules of team sports). By knowing what is developmentally appropriate, the professional can make suggestions on listening activities for parents to consider, when they express interest in auditory training and also in promoting age-appropriate life skills. For instance, when reminded that typical 10-year-olds can be relied on to get themselves up every morning with the aid of an alarm clock, parents of children with hearing loss might be interested in promoting that level of age-appropriate independence with assistive devices for their child.

2. *The Children's Home Inventory of Listening Difficulties (CHILD)*, developed by Anderson & Smaldino (2000), is a family-centered instrument designed to consider a range of listening and communication situations in the home environment. Fifteen scenarios are presented, to be rated on an 8-point scale. For example, the first item is this:

> Sit next to your child and look at a book together, or talk about something in front of you using familiar words and a normal conversational manner. Talk in a quiet place and sit so that you child is not looking at your face as you talk together. How difficult does it seem for your child to hear and understand what you say?

Parents rate their child's abilities as "great, good, okay but not easy, tough going," and so on. Other conditions to consider include speaking to the child in a quiet room without getting her attention first; listening abilities from the back seat of the car; hearing a clock radio alarm in the morning, and so on.

If old enough, children can complete a corresponding version as well (e.g., "You are sitting next to your mom or dad. You are looking at a book together or talking about something in front of you. You are not looking at mom's or dad's face as they talk to you. It's quiet. How difficult is it for you to hear and understand what they say?"). If differences between ratings occurs, an unknown problem has now been identified and can be more readily addressed. The *CHILD* provides a welcome opportunity to compare notes, problem-solve listening difficulties (discuss various assistive devices, increase practice on communication repair strategies, and so on) and fosters a sense of family ownership of both the problems and the solutions. The *CHILD* can also be used as a pre- and post-measure to evaluate the effects of a specific intervention.

3. *Time out! I didn't hear you* (Palmer, Butts, Lindley, & Snyder, 1996). If children express an interest in sports, concerns may arise about accommodations, safety, and legal access. This book provides family-friendly information to help make sports and sporting events accessible to children, and includes a chapter on role-model athletes with hearing loss.

4. *Self-advocacy skills for students who are deaf and hard of hearing* (English, 1997). When a child turns 15 or 16, he or she will be expected to participate in transition planning for post-high school settings. This curriculum covers the legal rights accorded a person with hearing loss both before and after high school, describes some basic "people skills" needed to speak up for oneself while not offending others, and includes role-playing and other practice strategies while encouraging the student to start developing a post-high school support system.

CHAPTER 4

Basic Counseling Skills: "Keeping the Door Open"

LEARNING OBJECTIVES

Readers of this chapter will be able to:

1. Describe four techniques to help "keep the door open" during the counseling process: monitoring proportions of "talk time," refraining from giving advice, surrendering the role of expert, and releasing conversational control.

2. Identify six listening strategies: minimal encouragers; paraphrasing; acknowledging and reflecting feelings; using "helping phrases" for clarification, providing feedback; and using silence as an opportunity for an individual to organize personal thoughts and feelings.

3. Describe the pitfalls of well-meaning reassurance and persuasion.

4. Give examples of psychological barriers to effective listening.

To Keep the Door Open

Chapter 3 described strategies to use as "door openers" in helping children with hearing impairment (and their parents) tell their stories. "Opening the door," however, is only the first step in the counseling process. The next steps are these:

- ☐ Help children tell their story
- ☑ Help them clarify their problem
- ☑ Help them challenge themselves to solve the problem
- ☐ Help them set a goal
- ☐ Help them develop an "action plan"

☐ Observe as they implement the plan
☐ Help them evaluate the plan

Although some glimpses of Steps 2 and 3 were seen earlier, this chapter will specifically focus on how to help children clarify their problem and how to help them challenge themselves to solve the problem.

During this process, we will see how easy it is for the wrong choice of words to effectively close the door that had been opened, and how the carefully worded response can keep the door open for as long as necessary to help with steps 2–7. Before looking at specific techniques, we need to consider four general principles to conducting a "counseling conversation": monitoring the proportion of "talk time," recognizing the effects of dispensing advice and assuming the role of expert, and the question of conversational control.

"Look Who's Talking"

It is a profoundly simple fact: only one person can talk at a time. The person who uses the most "talk time" is the person who is listened to the most. Ultimately, "keeping the door open" in counseling means being very careful not to dominate the talk time, but in fact, trying to talk as little as possible. This may be a common practice among adults interacting with other adults: we are accustomed to listening while a friend discusses a serious problem in great detail. We know in these circumstances we are not expected to say anything, just serve as a "sounding board." (As a reminder, a literal sounding board is a thin resonant board placed in a violin or piano, used to reinforce tones with sympathetic vibration. It does not produce any tones itself.)

Consideration of the proportion of talk time can be overlooked when adults communicate with children. Adults can be in the habit of immediately instructing children on what they need to do about their problem instead of finding out about what the child might want to do about the problem.

To demonstrate the effect of dominating "talk time," let's follow along with these two dialogues. Sarah, age 12, approaches us, sounding frustrated and annoyed:

SARAH: Do I have to wear these hearing aids all day?

ADULT: Yes, you do, otherwise you will fail all your classes. You could get them in a different color so you could hide them in your hair.

SARAH: Colors? Why would I want that?

ADULT: And don't forget to check those batteries.

You can almost hear the conversational door slamming in Sarah's face. Whatever she wanted to say, she was not given the chance, and in fact had even more reason than before to resent a decision made for her by someone else. Compare that dialogue to the following one:

SARAH: Do I have to wear these hearing aids all day?

ADULT: That's a problem?

SARAH: Oh yeah!!

ADULT: How so?

SARAH: It's really hard . . . the kids . . . Well, I'm OK in English class but then there is Eddie . . .

ADULT: Yeah? Eddie?

SARAH: Do you know Eddie? He's in my class but what a jerk, he tells everyone how dumb I am.

ADULT: Eddie says that?

SARAH: Yeah, I heard him talking to the speech teacher—can't hardly help hearing him!

ADULT: He's a loud mouth, that Eddie. Sounds like that hurt your feelings.

SARAH: Well, I don't think I'm dumb.

ADULT: There you go, you know what YOU are about. You mentioned English class?

SARAH: Well, the other kids don't wear hearing aids.

ADULT: Yeah.

SARAH: The teacher's great. . . . There's one kid, Shanique, she always sits next to me. . . . She tells me things I missed. And when I wear the hearing aids, she doesn't have to help so much. But when that Eddie is around . . .

ADULT: So you have a friend who helps you out and a kid who gives you grief.

SARAH: Yeah, I need to ignore that kid.

ADULT: And the other classes?

Many differences can be observed between these two dialogues, the most obvious being that the second dialogue was much longer

than the first. But what other differences between these two dialogues can we identify?

1. **Proportion of talk time.** In the first, the adult dominated the
   talk time. If we used a computer to obtain a word count, we would
   find that the adult used about 66 percent of the talk time, leaving little opportunity for the child to talk. In the second dialogue,
   the proportion reverses: the adult used only about 33 percent of
   the talk time, providing greater opportunity for Sarah to tell her
   story (as depicted in Figure 4.1).

Dialogue #1

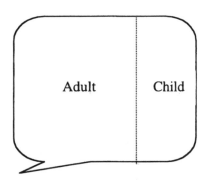

Dialogue #2

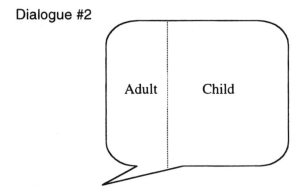

FIGURE 4.1 **"Look who's talking"**

It will be observed that during this extended talk time, Sarah also was able to clarify her problem and find the beginnings of a solution to her problem, but this did not happen by chance. The adult carefully chose words that would "keep the door open," a concept to be discussed later in the chapter.

The proportion of talk time was influenced by the adult's ability to "hear the knock" to an affective conversation. In the first dialogue, the adult did not pick up on the affective nature of the child's comment, and answered it as if it were only a request for information. This may have been an unrecognized communication mismatch, as described in Chapter 1, or possibly the adult felt the need to exert authority over the situation. Either way, Sarah was actively discouraged from expressing her point of view. Permitting the expression of an opposing point of view does not mean that the listener agrees with it, just that it is being attended to.

2. In the second dialogue, when the adult perceived the child was upset and angry, she **refrained from dispensing advice**. Her restraint paid off: by being given an indirect permission to "vent," Sarah had the opportunity to clarify her problem and come to her own conclusions about the situation. Sarah gets the chance to verbalize her self-perception as not being "dumb," as well as her need not to let Eddie bother her (challenging herself). She also hears herself saying that she is depending on a friend in English, although not as much as when using her hearing aids. If an adult pointed these things out, they would not be as revelatory as when she worked them out for herself. These realizations are consistent with Rogers' theory: that each person has the capacity to grow and find their own solutions, given a safe and supportive environment.

3. To keep the door open, the adult actively **surrendered the role of expert** on the basic question being addressed: What is it like to be Sarah right now? In all honesty, we have to acknowledge that in fact we don't truly know. It is often hard for adults to admit this, to say to a child, "I have no idea what it is like to be 12 years old with a hearing loss, please help me understand." But giving Sarah the opportunity to understand her own actions and motivations will help her move forward with a plan to effect a change.

4. **Conversational control.** One reason why the second dialogue evolved as far as it did was because the adult surrendered control of the conversation to the child. That is, the child talked about

what was on her mind, and was not sidetracked by other topics. The adult waited for topics and kept them "in the air" for as long as Sarah wanted to talk about them.

Following is an example of an unintentional "grabbing" for conversational control. This adult meets up with 17 year old Jorge for the first time in several months:

> **JORGE:**   Hi, Mr. Jacob, long time no see. I know, you're looking for my hearing aids, but I've decided to stop wearing them. Not only that, I've decided to leave school and get a job. I start at the mall on Monday.
>
> **MR. JACOBS:**   What do your friends say about this?

To his credit, although alarmed, Mr. Jacobs was trying not to rush in with unasked-for advice. But his response automatically narrowed the conversation to one consideration (friends' opinions), which may or may not have anything to do with the situation. There may be many things Jorge would have said here, but now his answer has to focus in on his friends. His decision may be about boredom with school, or falling grades, or family financial problems, or actually having no friends, but now we won't know. The door was not shut on him, but it was narrowed down to a topic that may or may not have been relevant. Limiting one's responses only to what has been said is called "verbal following" (Shames, 2000).

About Control: Who Owns This Hearing Loss?

Underlying each of these dialogues is a fundamental philosophical difference that can be addressed by how we answer this question, "Who owns this hearing loss?" In the first dialogue, the adult assumes she did. She answered with the authority of an expert and dictated actions that should be done. She did not give the child the freedom to express her concern, and provided answers that indicated that she "knew best." The counseling process could not continue because the adult did not help Sarah "challenge herself" as the person responsible for her hearing loss or her resulting interpersonal problems.

In the second dialogue, ownership of or responsibility for the hearing loss was accorded to the child. The adult here kept turning the conversation back to the child: What is your story, your perception? What do you want to do about it? Here the adult is helping Sarah challenge herself as capable of finding a solution (to "own" her hearing loss). The adult did not assume expertise about what it is like to be Sarah. She did not assume the responsibility of managing her personal objections with wearing hearing aids, but waited to see if Sarah would do so on her own. If the problem had been a technical one—such as interference with an FM system, feedback from a hearing aid, or confusion about a homework assignment—it would have "belonged" to the adult as part of the adult's area of expertise. The adult waited to find out first before proceeding, however, and then matched her responses accordingly.

When children have a hearing impairment, parents are the first "owners" or responsible parties, just as they are responsible for every aspect of their child's well-being and development. Over the course of time, parents face the task of transitioning ownership or responsibility of the hearing loss to the child, as he or she matures and becomes more able to manage his or her needs. By virtue of being involved with a family and child, however, professionals may unconsciously feel a sense of ownership, and inadvertently try to take over. Because this "take-over" is inappropriate, the family and later the child will resist, with passive-aggressive behaviors or open resentment—or, an equally undesired outcome, the family and/or child may become overly reliant, demonstrating a lack of independence. As with any other difficulty in life (a learning disability, an inability to control spending, problems with substance abuse, and so on), the persons experiencing the problem must "own" it in order to learn how to take care of it. Until they do, their ability to take care of their problem will be limited.

In the previous chapter, we explored strategies that might "open the door" to help a child tell his or her story. We then discussed four principles to consider while conducting a counseling conversation: (1) monitoring the proportion of "talk time," (2) recognizing the effects of dispensing advice, (3) surrendering the role of expert, and (4) releasing conversational control. We are now at the point where we need to consider this question: When we do talk, what should we say in order to keep the door open and advance the counseling process? This is a vital aspect of the counseling process, since every response we give influences the nature of the next comment from the child, and can advance, stall, or misdirect the intended outcomes. In order for us to know what to say, we have to first know what we are listening to. Following are some basic strategies to encourage conversation from the person we are listening to.

Basic Listening Skills: Not a Passive Process

There is a saying, "Easy listening exists only on the radio." At first listening may appear to be a very passive process but in fact, when done effectively, it is a highly active cognitive process, and requires one's full attention, a great deal of practice, and ongoing vigilance. Following is a description of six basic listening skills.

1. **Minimal encouragers**. These responses are the briefest of comments ("Uh-huh," "Really?", "Hmmm") and nonverbal behaviors (head nods, eye contact, leaning-in posture) that we use to let the speaker know we are paying attention. As mentioned earlier, Shames (2000) calls these behaviors *"verbal* followings," but of course our nonverbal reactions (body language, facial expressions) also "speak" this message. They come naturally to most people, but it is important to point out their positive effects in communication, and to appreciate the fact that we have the most basic of listening strategies in our repertoire already.

   An example of a minimal encourager is demonstrated in the second dialogue in response to the child's comment, "Other kids don't wear hearing aids." The adult could have explained that in fact thousands of children wear hearing aids across the country, but instead she let it go, surrendering the role of expert. "Yeah," in this environment, in this child's world, no one else wears hearing aids. The minimal encourager kept Sarah talking.

2. **Paraphrase**. As one would expect, this strategy attempts to sum up what was heard. Hearing oneself being paraphrased does not sound odd to the speaker; rather, it gives the message, "I am following along and I think I am getting your points." Refer back to the second dialogue, and you will find a paraphrase with this comment: "So you have a friend who helps you out and a kid who gives you grief." This comment did not put a halt to the child's contributions in the conversation, but actually helped her realize a solution to her problem: "Yeah, I need to ignore that kid."

3. **Acknowledge/reflect feelings.** This listening skill is often misunderstood to mean that one simply parrots back what one hears. A poor example might be this:

   "I hate it when it rains all weekend."
   "You're angry about the weather?"

In this instance, the speaker is not genuinely angry, just mildly annoyed or inconvenienced. The response, however, described an intense emotion that was not an accurate reflection of what was meant, so the first person is left to wonder what the second person is getting at.

A careful listener would try to acknowledge feelings when the feelings are apparently the heart of a problem. Humans experience strong emotions associated with loss, conflict, stress, uncertainty, and other difficult situations, and those emotions may be expressed overtly or subtly. Until the feelings are addressed, a person is not as likely to cope and problem-solve. The feelings are "in the way," and at the moment they are the more important issue. Talking to a carefully attentive listener helps a person see one's way through the difficulties and find some answers. Going back to a concept mentioned in Chapter 1, initially the "feeling mind" is interfering with the " "thinking mind," but once the interference is addressed, the "thinking mind" can be accessed (Goleman, 1995).

Reflecting feelings can be particularly important with children with hearing loss because they often lack the practice in labeling a feeling with a word. Difficulties in self-expression abound when one does not have the vocabulary to describe one's feelings. Remember the boy in Chapter 3 who comes home from school acting uncooperative and sullen. He is asked, "What's wrong?" and he responds, "I'm upset," but cannot go further because he can't explain what that means to him.

Egan (1998) suggests that in learning to become a nonprofessional counselor, we start reflecting feelings with a simple formulaic response, and once one's confidence and skills improve, we will feel comfortable in leaving the formula behind. After several exchanges between adult and child, the adult may find it helpful to say, "You feel . . . because. . . ." The blanks filled in are the emotions that are being expressed followed by the experiences or behaviors that the child is also describing. The second dialogue could have produced the following comment from an adult: "You feel upset because of what Eddie has been saying." Such a comment not only reflects feelings but summarizes as well.

Another example: If we think back to Curtis' circumstances, this response, "You're upset because you misunderstood another student," summarizes the situation but does not put any words in his mouth, and does not attempt to offer advice. Although a formulaic response is not routinely recommended, it may provide a starting point for persons new to personal adjustment counseling.

Taking the time to acknowledge feelings can be difficult for "professional problem solvers" such as teachers and other professionals. But doing so helps a child take things in the order of importance:

> What does it mean to acknowledge someone's feelings? It means letting the other person know that what they have said has made an impression on you, that their feelings matter to you, and that you are working hard to understand them. . . . It's tempting to jump over feelings. We want to get on with things, address the problem, to make everything better. We often seek to get feelings out of the way by fixing them. (Stone et al., 1999, p. 107)

4. **Use "Helping Phrases" for understanding.** Some "Helping Phrases" are offered below to use when we do or do not understand, but do want to keep the door open regardless to find out more. These are nonjudgmental, "tell me more, help me understand" types of phrases that might encourage a child to speak for him or herself.

"Helping Phrases" when you do understand:

It sounds like you feel . . .
You seem to be feeling . . .
My impression is . . . am I understanding you right?
The part that I understand is . . .
If I understand you right, you . . .

"Helping Phrases" when you do not understand:

The part that isn't clear to me is . . .
Could you tell me . . .?
Can you say more about . . .?
How is that for you?
How do you view that?
When do you feel that way?
How do you mean that?
I'm not clear on what you mean by . . .

What does that mean to you?
Is this what you're saying . . .?

Helping phrases can be found in the second dialogue: "Eddie says that?" "How so?" (tell me more), "You mentioned English class?"

5. **Provide feedback.** Giving feedback is a common practice in education: a teacher will return an essay with suggestions for the next revision, or children will offer suggestions to a classmate who gets stage fright when presenting an oral report. In counseling, feedback is more specifically meant as information on how one affects others. Frequently children are not fully aware of how they affect others, and feedback can help them keep their behavior on target and thus better achieve their goals. Following are some criteria for providing useful feedback (Long, 1996):

■ *Feedback is solicited rather than imposed*. By definition, feedback is a request for input. Adults will seek feedback from colleagues with a request to read a report for clarity and typographical errors. Job applicants will ask for feedback about the appearance of a resume or what to wear to an interview. If not solicited, comments can be considered suggestions, evaluations, or critiques, but not feedback.

This distinction is important to keep in mind: if an adult would like to provide feedback to a child, he or she will need to manage the situation so that the child can be in the position to request it. It is quite unlikely for a child to initiate the request for feedback, since he or she will probably not even know about the concept. A situation would need to be somewhat turned around so that the adult explains the process and makes the offer, in response to a child's concern, to provide feedback. To demonstrate this point, let us imagine that Martin has opened the door by mentioning to his teacher his difficulty making or keeping friends; the adult offers to conduct some low-profile observations and provide feedback, and the child accepts this offer:

MARTIN: I never have anyone to play with.

ADULT: Are you asking for some help?

MARTIN: Well. . . . like what?

ADULT: You could think about that and let me know. For example, I could stroll around during recess and lunch and see what goes on with your classmates. We could talk about it later, maybe figure out what's going on.

MARTIN: OK, that sounds good, just don't wave at me or anything.

The adult's feedback would then be directed to Martin's self-identified situation.

- *Feedback is descriptive rather than evaluative or judgmental.* Most people are aware that criticism is not part of the feedback process, since it can discourage a child from trying again. Interestingly, praise is as unhelpful as criticism in feedback: it doesn't provide any direction on how to grow. However, a neutral description of behaviors gives a child something to work with. The nature of these descriptions is addressed in the next point:

- *Feedback is specific rather than general.* An overall impression does not give much to work with, as with the observation, "You didn't spend much time playing with any particular child in recess." The description of specific events are more meaningful; for example, "You seemed to hear Fred's comment about the lunch choices today but you didn't answer him—it might have seemed to him that you were ignoring him," or "You seemed pretty angry about what Carlos said about your new sneakers, but it sounded like a joke to me, is that possible? How would we know the difference?" These comments are focused on communication breakdowns, but other social decisions or reactions might also be observed and described: "The team decided to change the rules for that game, and you refused to agree so you left the game by yourself. I guess you had a problem with this?"

- *Feedback is checked to ensure clear communication.* All the examples above provide not only a description of the behavior or event, but a check on accuracy: Is that how it seemed to you? Without this last criterion, we would effectively close the door instead of keeping it open. Clearly, feedback must be presented as topics to explore further, rather than a checklist of behaviors with no further discussion. A child cannot be expected to work out solutions to these problems entirely on his or her own. If he or she knew how, there wouldn't be problems to begin with.

6. **Silence.** Not speaking may not seem like a very helpful response, and in our Western culture, we are often uncomfortable with the suggestion to refrain from speaking for more than a few seconds. However, silence can give a child time to organize his or her thoughts on a topic that may be unfamiliar ground, or difficult to talk about. It can also be a way of acknowledging the difficulty a child is going through at that moment. In other words, when one feels, "I don't know what to say," then perhaps "no words" is the right thing to offer.

Following are some excerpts from some writers who have thought about the effects of silence:

> Silence is an important component of any therapeutic relationship. . . . reflective silence invariably follows some emotionally, laden material. This silence is a time out to think about and to experience the feelings that have been brought to the surface. . . . (Luterman, 1996, p. 102)

> Periods of silence during a conversation are very acceptable within some cultures (e.g., the Arabic culture), but less acceptable in others. In the general United States, silences during conversation can be disconcerting, particularly when two parties are just getting acquainted . . . Unfortunately, many people's inclination is to say something to break a silence; often, this is the worst thing to do. . . . There are some limitations to silence. Silences that last much longer than about 5 seconds (e.g., 10–15 seconds) are likely to be terminated by the interviewer, and result in shorter verbalizations from interviewees." (Shipley, 1997, pp. 69–70)

> What does it mean to listen to a voice before it has spoken? It means making space for the other, honoring the other. It means not rushing in to fill [others'] silence with fearful speech of our own and not coerce them into saying things we want to hear. It means entering into [another's] world so that he or she perceives you as someone who has the promise of being able to hear another person's truth. (Palmer, 1998, p. 46)

An adult typically does not set out with a plan to intentionally maintain silence when interacting with a child. This concept is presented here as another response to consider, and to not shy away from if it seems it might help the child talk further.

Summary of Basic Listening Skills

The previous section described these six listening skills:

- Minimal encouragers and "verbal followings"
- Paraphrasing
- Acknowledging and reflecting feelings
- Using "helping phrases"
- Providing feedback
- Silence

It is suggested that professionals attempt to improve one skill at a time, rather than try to develop a broad range of listening skills all at once and then risk discouragement when the learning becomes difficult. The above skills are roughly in order of difficulty—for instance, most readers will realize that they already provide minimal encouragers. If that is the case, the next task to consider is to evaluate how effective these are in keeping the door open to a conversation.

The following section will describe two communication efforts that would appear to help keep the door open but in fact are more likely to close it at least partway. These are *reassurance* and *persuasion*.

Two Common Pitfalls in Counseling

Reassurance. It seems to be part of human nature, certainly among helping professionals, to eagerly reassure individuals that they should not be upset or worried or unhappy, regardless of the situation. The motive behind this act probably is an altruistic attempt to reduce anxiety so that others will feel better. However, as Clark (1994) points out, these comments only make the *speaker* feel better. While attempting to ease a person's mind, the speaker actually is conveying this message: "You should not be feeling what you feel right now. You are too upset to see things as I do, and how I see them is far more accurate. You think you are having problems, but you really aren't." Let's follow this conversation between Curtis and his father to consider the effects of inappropriate reassurance:

CURTIS: Dad, I really blew it today. I misunderstood another kid about track practice and overreacted. I kinda pushed him against the wall. I feel like such a jerk.

DAD: I'm sure he realized you have a hearing loss. He's probably already forgotten about it.

Curtis is left with little to say after that, unless he wanted to argue his point of view. Feeling upset, he opened a door to talk it over with his father, but his father unintentionally closed it fast. His father was trying to take the sting out of the event, but by downplaying the situation, he is telling Curtis that although he thought this was important, it was not. Instead of letting him know, "I'm trying to understand how you feel," the father is saying, "You read the situation all wrong, you have no right to feel like this." From Curtis' point of view, he is likely to feel confused rather than understood: "I told you something serious and you discounted it. It still feels serious, even though you think it isn't, and now I can't even talk about it with you."

Compare the above to the following version, where the father refrains from reassurance in order to keep the door open:

CURTIS: Dad, I really blew it today. I misunderstood another kid about track practice and overreacted. I kinda pushed him against the wall. I feel like such a jerk.

DAD: Now I know why you were looking so down. What all happened?

CURTIS: [provides the details]

DAD: That's a tough situation. Have you decided what to do?

Let's look at another example of inappropriate reassurance. This time, let's imagine Martin confiding to his teacher:

MARTIN: Ms. M., it feels like the kids here are avoiding me.

MS. M.: That's not true! Remember how Barbara helped you with that story last week?

As Stone and his colleagues (1999) say, as with other affective conversations, Martin's comment is not about what is true, it is about what is important. What is important at this moment was Martin's feelings of loneliness, but Ms. M. did not acknowledge them—instead, she denied them by providing empty words of consolation. Martin could follow her response by arguing his point, but he probably already regrets expressing his thoughts, and is not likely to continue onward.

As we did before with Curtis, let's revisit this conversation and instead of having the teacher dispense reassurance, have her keep the door open:

> **MARTIN:** Ms. M., it feels like the kids here are avoiding me.
>
> **MS. M.:** I didn't know you felt this way, Martin.
>
> **MARTIN:** Well, it's not all the time, but it happens so much, it's hard to be sure.
>
> **MS. M:** Hard to be sure?
>
> **MARTIN:** About what the kids think of me. I want to be, ya know, with them, like everyone else.
>
> **MS. M:** It doesn't feel that way right now?
>
> **MARTIN:** Most of the time, no. . . .

And so on. Ms. M. kept the door open by giving Martin all the room he needed to say what is hard to talk about (feeling unpopular, wanting things to be different).

Sometimes reassurance is quite valid, as when one wants to verify a factual situation:

> **PERSON A:** I think I forgot to turn off the TV before we left the house.
>
> **PERSON B:** Don't worry, I checked everything, including the TV. It's definitely off.

Feelings were not involved in Person A's comment, and Person B provided reassurance so that Person A would not need to continue wondering about this fact. When talking to Curtis and Martin, the adults did not eliminate the need to keep wondering, but instead got the children worrying even more: Why did you not hear what I just said?

When considering inappropriate reassurance, we need to look again at the question of control. By attempting to reassure the child in question, both adults were trying to control the children's reaction or perception, instead of acknowledging that what they felt was legitimate. Lundberg and Lundberg (1995) have written a book that focuses entirely on the inadvertent effects of reassurance. In *I Don't Have to Make Everything All Better*, their first principle is, "Let me feel what I am feeling." Adults may find it hard to let this occur, and may worry that to do so would be to lose control over the situation.

Persuasion. Luterman (1996) describes another aspect of "counseling-gone-wrong," which he calls "counseling by persuasion." He asks professionals to challenge their reasons for persuading an individual to "see it their way." He writes:

> The underlying assumption of this approach is that "I as a professional have all of this information and experience. You as the client are ignorant of so many things that you need to know; therefore, I can make a better decision for you than you can for yourself. . . ." This mode of counseling assumes that [clients] are weak and are incapable of effective decision making. . . . (p. 4)

When a professional is in "persuasion mode," by definition he or she is talking and therefore not listening. More than just a door-closer, however, persuasion takes away an opportunity for a parent or child to determine one's own mind and to assume ownership of the situation. For example, parents who are persuaded to use a particular communication strategy (sign language, oral/aural communication, cued speech, or others) that they don't really prefer, are not committed to the decision and are not likely to follow through on its implementation. Why should they? After all, it was someone else's decision, not what they really wanted to do. In such a circumstance, parents engage in an unspoken struggle for control, but lose to the professional whose advice carries the day. Professionals may insist on "being right" (discussed again later), yet there is no objective evidence of what is "right" for a particular family. In fact, the "right" course of action is the one the family decides will fit their lives best, and what they want to work for. Listen to this ongoing struggle with "being right" professionals as described by this parent:

> No one in my family knew anything about deafness before our son was born. We are from India, and there are cultural reasons why we are not comfortable with learning sign language, so we decided on a cochlear implant. We find ourselves always defending our decision to people who really have no involvement in our lives, but somehow feel they

have the right to tell us we did the wrong thing. How can they possibly know that? What right do they have to say these things? Yet because they are so adamant, and because his progress is a little slow, I often worry, what if they are right?

This family was honest with itself and knew what it wanted to do. Instead of providing support to work through ongoing difficulties, professionals were causing the parents to doubt themselves and were still trying to persuade them of what they *should have done*—what could be less helpful than that? This mother poses a fundamental question: What right does a professional have to persuade a family against its wishes? Once all professionals provide all relevant information possible to make an informed decision, the family has every right to decide their future. Once again, we are looking at the issue of control.

This same line of reasoning can be extended to the pediatric population as well. A child who is persuaded to follow our recommendations does not take full ownership of his or her hearing problems; obeying someone else is not accepting personal responsibility. Imagine a professional saying to a child, "You really need to wear those hearing aids in all your classes. Let's arrange a deal: if you wear them every day this week, I'll have a pizza delivered at lunchtime on Friday." If the child complies, it's to earn the pizza, not because she has identified her listening problems and has decided to be responsible for helping herself. Persuasion results in what Clark (1994) calls an unbalanced relationship which "can be detrimental to successful hearing care" (p. 19). To lead a child to self-sufficiency, a model of "mutual participation" must be developed in the child-adult relationship. Using persuasion is not mutual, only one-way and coercive.

Barriers to Listening: How Does the Door Slam Shut?

Keeping the door open relies more on listening than on talking. Remember how in the second dialogue, the listener used relatively little of the "talk time," allowing the child to use most of it. Unfortunately, as important as it is, listening carefully is a harder task than talking. Parsons (1995) explains that careful listening requires practice, since we are by nature "imperfect listeners."

Several psychological barriers interfere with listening effectively. Among the most insidious barriers is *habituation*, whereby we stop reacting to comments that are presented very frequently. Professionals quickly lose track of the number of times they hear a child insist that he or she can manage without hearing aids or cochlear implant, for instance. When one begins to operate under the assumption that this story is the same one heard countless times before, one stops listening to the individual trying to "get through" at that moment—a very strong barrier has been erected.

Other "Barriers to Listening" include:

- *Competing with the Speaker*. "Competing" in this sense means the habit of developing a self-conversation about our own impressions of what we hear, rather than fully tuning in to the speaker's actual words ("This sounds like a classic sense of denial" or, "He's having the same problems as the student who came in here this morning"). During this process, we are actually listening to ourselves, not the speaker. Once that occurs, we are not capable of keeping the door open because we haven't been following the speaker's words carefully enough to know what to say next.
- *Hearing with Filters*. As with the example above, this behavior involves a "turning inward," responding to one's own experiences and emotional reactions while the speaker presents his or her story. Because we ourselves are not devoid of emotional reactions, and because we cannot suppress the memory of our experiences, this barrier is a difficult one to avoid, especially because it usually shows up unexpectedly and catches us off guard. The important point is that we recognize it is happening and be aware of its potential as a barrier.
- *Day Dreaming*. This barrier is partly affected by habituation, and partly by our usual press for time: can I multitask while listening to this speaker, in order to take care of other responsibilities at the same time? The answer is, simply, no. Keeping the door open with careful attention is a full-time cognitive task. Less than full attention is easily perceived by the speaker, and he or she will feel the door gradually close (Figure 4.2).
- *Identifying*. "The same thing happened to me!" This response is intended to help the speaker feel he or she is not alone. However, it actually has a very different and almost confusing effect. Imagine

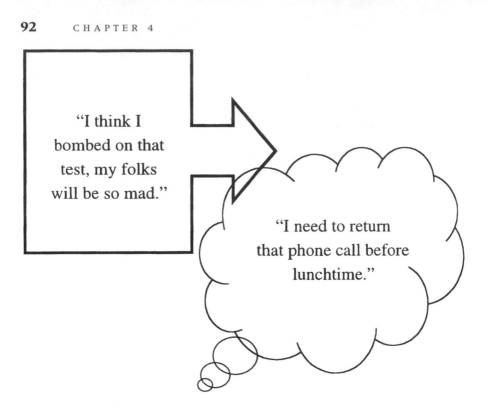

FIGURE 4.2   Day dreaming is a barrier to listening

seeing a student after a summer vacation, and asking how she is doing. She responds, "I'm kinda shaky right now, my favorite uncle died suddenly last month." We respond, "I know how you're feeling, I've lost loved ones, too." If we go back to the idea from Chapter 3 about the spotlight metaphor (Stone et al. 1999), we have effectively stepped into the spotlight and are asking the student to share it with us. And if we are hoping to keep the door open, we have made that less likely, because we are asking her now to think about the losses in **our** lives. This does not help her at all, it only confuses the situation. "I would like to talk about my uncle, but now I have to think about you, too." What is needed right now is to keep the spotlight solely on her: "I am so sorry. You said it was sudden?" This kind of response keeps the door wide: if she wants to talk more, she can hear the invitation, and the conversation is focused only on her.

■ *Being Right.* This barrier may be one of the most difficult to overcome, because, for the most part, professionals *are* right. We saw an example of Being Right in the first dialogue: "Yes, you do have to wear the hearing aids all day, otherwise you will fail school." The door slams shut! There is nothing left for the child to say except complain, argue, or express resentment. The listener may have been trying to keep the door open, but instead created a barrier with a communication mismatch: The child is expressing a personal adjustment concern, and the professional is providing an informational answer.

Professionals feel ethically responsible for Being Right, and with regard to providing professional support (technology, instruction, grading, testing), Being Right can be accurately interpreted as providing the best support possible, keeping current with research, and so on. But we don't want to confuse these responsibilities with personal adjustment concerns. These concerns have no right or wrong position, and do not require us to take a stand on them. They belong to the speaker, and if we insist on Being Right, we take over a problem that does not belong to us.

This section described several barriers to listening. Now that we are aware of them, what do we do about them? Once a barrier has been named and described, readers may quickly realize which ones have been part of their listening behaviors. As with other interpersonal skills, awareness is the first and most important step; once a professional is aware that an insistence for "being right," or habituating, or identifying with the speaker could pose potential barriers to listening, he or she can actively self-monitor and practice replacing a barrier with full attention and careful following of the speaker's concerns. Improving one's listening skills is a lifetime endeavor, but the results are worth the effort.

"Back to Cases"

In Chapter 3, we looked at how to open the door to a counseling conversation with a child (or parent), and in this chapter we considered ways to keep the door open in order to help a child clarify a problem and challenge him or herself to address the problem. Let us return to the children first presented in Chapter 1—Fatima, Martin, and Curtis—

and attempt to use these listening strategies as a way to provide counseling support for their personal adjustment problems.

Fatima

We will recall that Fatima is becoming withdrawn and is losing weight. There is no question, something is very much on her mind. However, she has not opened the door herself—that is, she has not mentioned anything of consequence for her teacher to respond to, and she has not been forthcoming to general queries such as "How are you doing these days, Fatima?" Her teacher is worried and wants to help, so she decides to try out the *I Start/You Finish* activity as a door-opener. She asks Fatima to stay behind for a couple minutes when class is dismissed for lunch.

TEACHER: Fatima, I found an interesting idea the other day, and was wondering if you could help me try it out. It works like this: I start a sentence, and you finish it. Wanna try it with me?

FATIMA: I guess so, sure.

TEACHER: Good, thanks. Here's the first one: "I am happy when . . ." How would you finish that one?

FATIMA: (long pause) Well, I guess when I play with my cats and dog.

TEACHER: I didn't know you have pets. (helping phrase: "tell me more")

FATIMA: (becomes animated) Yeah, the cats are named Blackie and Whitey, and the dog is named Elvis. My dad likes to say, "Elvis has left the building" when we let him outside. It always makes him laugh for some reason.

TEACHER: So you really like your pets. (paraphrasing)

FATIMA: They're the best pets a kid could have.

TEACHER: OK, let's try the next one. Here we go: "I am sad when . . ."

FATIMA: (nods but does not answer)

TEACHER: (carefully) How would you answer that one?

FATIMA: I am sad when . . . my mom cries.

TEACHER: Your mom cries?

FATIMA: Well, I think so, it looks like it. My grandma, she's really sick, everyone tries not to talk about it when I'm around but I think maybe she is dying. She's in the hospital and my mom is always there. When she comes home, she looks awful, like she is crying all the time. But she keeps telling me everything is OK.

TEACHER: Your grandmother is really sick? And your mom is so sad. (paraphrasing) I didn't know.

FATIMA: (looks away, does not answer)

TEACHER: This sentence thing helped me understand that you are worried and sad, too, maybe. (reflecting/acknowledging feelings)

FATIMA: (nods) I pretend I don't know, maybe that will help my mom.

The teacher has helped Fatima tell her story and clarify her concerns. She also found out that Fatima already understands the situation quite well and has accepted the challenge of trying to help (by pretending ignorance).

Since the teacher is finding out what is going on, she would not pursue the other incomplete sentences, since the second one opened the door to the personal adjustment concern. It's just as possible that this particular incomplete sentence might not have uncovered a difficulty; perhaps the others might get to very different concerns:

The thing I like most about the world is. . . .

my dad reading to me at bedtime.
when my mom isn't on business trips.
spending the night with my best pal.

The one thing in the world I would most like to change would be . . .

getting a little sister.
not needing hearing aids.
my dad finding a job.

Because I have a hearing loss . . .

I don't have any friends.
I can't use the phone like my friends do.
I keep making mistakes, it's embarrassing.

The obvious point is, we don't know what the answers are going to be. In our example above, the teacher may have first thought that Fatima's stress was associated with having a hearing loss, but finds out it is from a very different family circumstance. Now that she knows, she is better equipped to decide if she should proceed as a nonprofessional counselor, or make a referral to a (professional) school counselor.

Note that the teacher did not provide reassurance ("Everything is going to be OK, you'll see") or try to make her feel better ("You're being a brave little girl").

Martin

We came to know Martin as a youngster who seemed alone in a room full of peers. Little is known about him: is he shy, insecure, uncomfortable with being "different"? His school speech-language pathologist has been watching and waiting to see if Martin will open the door, but he is not forthcoming. She decides to try out the *CPR Scale* to see if it will help both of them talk about social relationships.

SLP: Martin, this morning, instead of our usual speech work, I wanted to use this little game, to help us talk about school and things. I'll read the words in each box, and your job is to make a check in the box that fits you best. Here's a pencil—ready? The first one says, (1) I like school. (2) School is OK. (3) I don't like school. Which one describes how you feel?

M: (silently checks, School is OK).

SLP: School is OK for you? (He nods. She waits, and he starts to add something, then changes his mind.)

SLP: Let's look at the next one. (1) I have some good friends in school. (2) I have one good friend in school. (3) I don't have good friends in school. Which one describes you, Martin?

M: (he puts down the pencil). The last one. I don't have any friends in school at all.

SLP: (picks up the pencil and marks the last box.) Oh.

M: Like I'm invisible or something. Kids talk right over me. I hate that.

SLP: That sounds lonely. (reflecting feelings) (He looks unsure, and she explains the word.)

M: Lonely, yeah, maybe.

SLP: (She waits, thinking he is getting closer to talking. She decides to skip to #4). Well, let's see about this one. We have: (1) Mostly, other kids like me. (2) Sometimes, other kids don't like me. (3) Other children don't really like me.

M: (looks down, doesn't answer).

SLP: This can be hard to talk about. (helping phrase)

M: (not seeming to hear her) Kids don't either like me or not like me, they just don't do nothing with me.

SLP: Oh.

M: Yeah, they play that ball game outside, I don't know what that is, and then when they're done, they hang out by the front and goof around, kinda pushing each other around like they're being mean but they're laughing. I don't know . . .

SLP: You don't know. . . . (he shrugs). Sounds like you would like to do those things too.

M: (getting angry) I WOULD! I would like to be . . . with the guys.

SLP: You want to be better at being with other kids, talking with them and playing with them. (paraphrase)

M: Yeah. . . .

The SLP was almost sure that Martin would prefer to be "with the guys," but if she had put the words in his mouth, he might have denied that he was having any problems. Using the *CPR Scale*, the SLP opened the door by giving him the opportunity to clarify his problem and his desire to change the situation. The counseling process can now advance toward goal setting and developing a plan for change (described in Chapter 5).

Curtis

Finally, we return to Curtis, a teen who jumped to conclusions and is mortified about how he overreacted. His first instinct was to drop off the team to avoid seeing his teammate again, but he is also mad at himself with this tentative decision, feeling very disappointed about missing out on track. Let's imagine that he keeps an appointment with his school audiologist, who can't help but see that he is very unhappy.

AUD: Curtis, you look miserable. Can I help at all?

C: No, I blew it big time and now everything is ruined. (He explains everything, including his plan to leave the team.)

AUD: Well, that's one idea. There may be others.

C: Like what? Like apologizing? No way.

AUD: (doesn't answer)

C: I mean, just thinking about that freaks me out.

AUD: Apologizing makes you nervous.

C: (kicks the table leg) I really like track, too.

AUD: Yeah.

C: If I apologize, he'll laugh at me, call me a jerk.

AUD: Hmm.

C: (sounding abandoned) I hardly even know the guy! It's not like apologizing to a friend. With my old friends at my old school, I could do that and be OK, they understood. Here, I don't know.

AUD: You're trying to decide if track is worth it.

C: Yeah.

AUD: Is there another way of thinking about this? Like not only is there apologizing, there is also explaining: you could explain that it's hard to hear in noisy hallways, and you don't have any friends yet so you don't know what people are thinking.

C: Those things are true, that's for sure.

AUD: Since they are true, they might not be too hard to explain.

C: Yeah, I could probably explain those things.

AUD: When I'm trying to understand what someone is deciding, I draw a line like this (draws) and put numbers from one to ten at the ends. If we were to say, one means, "No way am I gonna talk to this guy," and 10 means, "I am completely ready," where would you be right now?

C: Maybe a 5. Or a 6.

AUD: (nods) Half-way sure, then.

C: (shakes his head, stares out the window)

The audiologist could tell Curtis did not really want to drop out of track but could not come up with an alternative at first. To take the pressure off the prospect of apologizing, the audiologist provided another scenario, one that was still honest but not as intimidating. In addition to using the *Readiness Scale* to help Curtis consider doing something difficult, the audiologist was using the Rational Emotive Behavior Approach (REBT) described in Chapter 3. He heard Curtis express *absolutes* (i.e., the only solution was to drop off the team) and he suggested that Curtis reframe that into at least one other possibility.

In the next chapter, we will advance the counseling process to its conclusion: to decide whether to refer, or to help a child set a goal and practice problem solving.

Chapter Summary

- Several practices were offered as strategies to "keep the door open" once a child or parent begins a conversation.
- A challenge for professionals is to decide how to answer the question, "Who owns this hearing loss?" If they find themselves solving a child's personal adjustment problems, chances are they believe they own the loss to some extent.
- Basic listening skills were described and shown to be active rather than passive activities. Two pitfalls to listening were also described, as well a set of "listening barriers."
- Example conversations with our case studies and the use of different self-assessment instruments demonstrated ways to "keep the door open."

Learning Activities

Clarification Activity

With a learning partner, describe:

- How you might try to monitor the amount of talk time used
- How you might remember to avoid giving advice
- How you might attempt to release conversational control

Modeling Activity

With a learning partner, develop a role-playing scenario to present to others, using this comment as an opener (from Chapter 3): Sarah, age 12, says, "No one else in school wears hearing aids." One partner will take the part of Sarah and the other partner the role of an adult. Together, develop a short script that will demonstrate to your audience these listening strategies: minimal encouragers, paraphrasing, acknowledging and reflecting feelings, using helping phrases, and using silence. Perform your scene and then moderate a discussion about the nature of the conversation that ensued by applying these strategies.

Writing Activity

Write a paragraph identifying the easiest aspect to developing the scenario above, and also the one hardest aspect. Are these related to personality or to learning?

Practice/Feedback

Following are comments first presented in the Learning Activities in Chapter 3. Now that we are better equipped to "keep the door open," practice responding to these comments with a learning partner, and ask the partner to carry on an exchange for a couple minutes. For instructional purposes, intentionally use (1) inappropriate reassurance, (2) persuasion, and/or (3) a "being right" response. What happened to the conversation?

- *Mr. Bonito, parent:* "For the first time in her short life, Dina was scoring at the top of a scale instead of the bottom on some therapy goals. Things seemed to be looking up, and then we heard our insurance claim was denied. We owe over $1,000 now."

- *Mrs. Clemson, parent:* "I love Michael, of course, but if I had known sooner that he was deaf, I wouldn't have had a second child— she's deaf too."
- *Samantha, age 14:* "I think I bombed on that test, my parents will be so mad."

Completing the Counseling Process: Goals, Plans, and Intervention

LEARNING OBJECTIVES

Readers of this chapter will be able to:

1. Describe the final steps in completing the counseling process.
2. Provide a rationale for providing intervention in social skills and emotional self-awareness.
3. Describe a set of materials available for the nonprofessional counselor.
4. Create a referral system for their community.

We can see from our checklist that we are progressing through the counseling process:

☐ Help children tell their story
☐ Help them clarify their problem
☐ Help them challenge themselves to solve the problem
☑ Help them set a goal
☑ Help them develop an "action plan"
☑ Observe as they implement the plan
☑ Help them evaluate the plan

The material in the first part of this chapter will feel like familiar territory to most readers, since professionals are accomplished goal setters and plan developers. Consequently, relatively little time will be spent here examining these steps. In keeping with the philosophy that the child owns or has responsibility for the hearing loss, as well as the problems that occur as a result of having a hearing loss, we will promote the child's ability also to own the solutions to the problems, by helping the child actively develop goals and test plans. Since the problem belongs to the child, he or she will learn how to find a solution only if given the opportunity. Therefore, the challenge here will be "helping" rather than "taking over." In sports parlance, we will strive not to "take the ball and run with it" because the ball belongs to the child.

"Back to Cases"

Fatima

Fatima's teacher has learned that a beloved family member is very ill, but no one is discussing it with Fatima. Now that she knows the situation, the teacher feels the concern of professional boundaries. It seems like Fatima needs help talking to her mother, but bringing this to the mother's attention may not be very helpful, since the mother also seems to need help talking to Fatima. The problem at hand felt "bigger" than the teacher was comfortable with, so she knew a referral to the school counselor was in order. We rejoin them as she brings up this option to Fatima.

> **TEACHER:**   This sentence game helped me understand that you are worried and sad, too, maybe.
>
> **FATIMA:**   (nods) I pretend I don't know, maybe that will help my mom.
>
> **TEACHER:**   Pretending not to know may or may not help your mom, Fatima, I just don't know about that. I do know someone who might, though—remember Mrs. Campbell? She dropped in our class the other day to say hi.
>
> **FATIMA:**   Sure, she had a lot of books she said we could read.
>
> **TEACHER:**   She is great at helping children when they are sad and worried like you are. I'd like to walk with you down to her office and introduce you, and ask you to tell her what you just shared with me. Would you be comfortable doing that? She is a good listener and she may be able to help you and your mom talk about your grandma.
>
> **FATIMA:**   OK, I like her enough. I want to help my mom, mainly, so we can go now if you want.

This counseling conversation was a highly effective start to helping Fatima with her problem. The teacher was able to help Fatima confide about a secret she was carrying, and then seek out professional support so that she could handle it in a more healthy fashion. Because the topics of her grandmother's illness and her mother's sadness are no longer taboo for Fatima, she may be more likely to open the door herself when she is burdened with another concern in the future.

The next two scenarios take us through some goal setting and the development of action plans for Martin and Curtis. Of course we are fully aware that there is no guaranteed strategy for any one individual, and that there are individual differences to problem solving, influenced by situation, personality, experience, and even gender (Murphy & Ross, 1987; Ronning, McCurdy, & Ballinger, 1984). But if the child assumes responsibility for goals and plans, it is highly likely that these will be congruent with his or her personal interests and therefore more likely to be achieved.

Martin

When we left Martin, he was talking to the speech-language pathologist about watching other boys in school play together, and expressing interest in joining them. Now that he has clarified his problem, she would like to help him accept the challenge of solving the problem:

> **SLP:** You want to be better at being with other kids, talking with them and playing with them.
>
> **M:** Yeah . .
>
> **SLP:** There are some things you could learn about that.
>
> **M:** (skeptical) Like what?
>
> **SLP:** There are "friend" skills you could learn, just like you are learning speech and math and reading. It takes practice like everything else, but it sounds like it's important to you, and you would be OK with practicing. What do you think?
>
> **M:** (looks doubtful but a little hopeful, too) That would be OK, sure.

The speech-language pathologist is leading Martin to the step in identifying an initial goal. He had mentioned a general desire to join the group of boys at recess, but that seems a little too "advanced" as a first step.

SLP: Is there one boy you would say is extra nice or friendly? One boy you would like to be with and comfortable with?

M: Yeah, there's Keith, he is kinda like me, you know, like . . . quiet.

SLP: (nods) He sounds like someone you could talk to, hang out with. Can you think of a goal to start out with?

M: What do you mean, goal?

SLP: (she realizes she needs to back up, so she explains, shows him the sign for goal). Something you "shoot for," or want to accomplish, like collecting every baseball card from your favorite team, or reading a book by yourself. You had a goal last summer, remember? You told me you wanted to be able to swim across the deep end of the pool, so you took lessons and you did it. You didn't use the word "goal," but that's what it was.

M: Something to shoot for . . . you mean, like how I want a new skateboard? So my mom says I have to save my allowance, and when I have half the money, she would pay half too—like that?

SLP: That's it, your goal is to own the skateboard, and saving the money is your plan. Before, your goal was to swim the deep end, so your plan was to take swimming lessons.

M: I need a plan for making friends, then?

In order to keep his thinking and word use straight, the speech-language pathologist pulls out paper and pencil and draws a target or bull's eye on the right hand side (Figure 5.1)

SLP: Here is your first goal, from what I can tell: become friends with one boy, Keith, am I right?

M: Yeah. That would be good.

SLP: So your plan for that (she draws a long arrow aiming at the target) would be, what? What kinds of things would help you get there?

M: (looks at her blankly, helplessly)

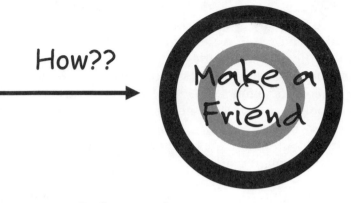

FIGURE 5.1   Goal versus plan

The speech-language pathologist can think of several suggestions and is strongly inclined to explain them, but wants to promote Martin's problem-solving skills above the sake of expediency. She waits and becomes fairly sure that Martin does not know how to proceed.

> **SLP:**   Martin, the thing is, I don't know what it's like to be an 8-year old boy. I could make suggestions, but I could make mistakes about it. It looks like the thing to do is for you to think about this, watch other kids. Like being an investigator in that book your read, those boys who solved mysteries.
>
> **M:**   (looking discouraged) One thing they do, they talk all the time. It's too fast, and all at once, I can't figure it out.
>
> **SLP:**   That's another thing I don't know about: having a hearing loss like you do. You just described a big problem when there is a group of boys, and we can talk later about how you can come up with a plan for that. Let's stick with our first goal, and later we will get to the rest. The first goal was to be friends with Keith (points to the target). I'd like you to think of a plan for that (points to the arrow) and tell me tomorrow.

The speech-language pathologist was determined to keep the ball in Martin's court. She also wanted to provide a deadline so that Martin would not stall or put off the task. Martin looked unsettled by the prospect but the next day he approached her in the hall, looking very animated:

M: You know how you put kids together to do writing work? And how you usually put me with Jessica? Could you put me with Keith? And while we do our work, I could ask him to come to my house on Saturday to play video games. I know he likes them and I heard him say he doesn't have the kind I do. But when you do put us together, it needs to be at the table near the book corner so I can hear him. Usually with Jessica, you give her the FM but I don't want to use that right away with Keith. I'll ask him to look at me when he talks, and show him how this implant works.

The speech-language pathologist was almost speechless! She did not expect him to have developed his plan to such detail. She realized he knew the conditions he needed to break the ice, and now he could use her as a facilitator. From this point on, the speech-language pathologist stays involved in his goal setting and plan development. It becomes a theme within her therapy time as well, using "Friendship Coaching" as a framework (described in the next section). The last step in the counseling process, helping Martin evaluate his plans, will also be part of "speech time." Martin is on his way to learning how to break through the impasse he had been facing.

Curtis

Unlike Martin, Curtis has already established a goal: to avoid further embarrassment. But the audiologist hears that Curtis is torn: his response to the *Readiness Scale* shows his uncertainty, and his desire to stay on the track team is also a goal.

AUD: If I drew a line here, and put numbers from one to ten, one meaning "No way am I gonna talk to this guy," and 10 meaning "I am completely ready," where would you be right now?

C: Maybe a 5. Or a 6.

AUD: (nods) Halfway sure, then.

C: (shakes his head, stares out the window)

AUD: The thing is, you don't have to make a decision right away.

C: Yeah, I know. There's no rush or anything.

AUD: (waits)

c: I wish this had never happened. I love track.

AUD: Yeah.

c: But it did happen and now I'm stuck.

AUD: You could stay stuck or you could find a way to get un-stuck. To get unstuck, it always helps to figure out a goal. One goal would be to avoid this kid, like you said. But you had an-other goal before, to be on the track team. Is one canceling out the other?

c: No, I want both as goals. But I know what you're saying, I need to choose.

AUD: On this scale, you thought you were at 5 or 6. What would you need to do to make it maybe an 8?

c: (shrugs) I could just go to practice, see what happens.

AUD: You could do that.

c: (sighs deeply) I could see if that guy is still mad at me. Maybe talk to him.

AUD: You could do that, too.

The audiologist does not think Curtis needs further assistance in work-ing out his problem. He prioritized his goals, and the plan to achieve the primary goal was self-evident. In addition, he had the social skills necessary to negotiate the apology. His first reaction did not have to end up being his last one, because the adult listener gave him the chance to find his way, without offering advice.

Note in both of these counseling conversations, control was left with the child: "What do you want to do? How do you want to do it?" In more complex situations, the adult would also want the child to de-termine, "How will you know if it worked?" Because the adult gives the child guided practice and the opportunity to be actively engaged in the process, the child's repertoire of important problem-solving skills is improved (Gange, 1980).

Providing Intervention

Throughout this book, we have considered a range of possibilities that might account for the problems demonstrated by children presented as case studies in Chapter 1. It was speculated that perhaps Fatima was developing some self-consciousness about being the only child in her school with a hearing loss, but it was ultimately learned that there was something very serious (though unrelated to hearing loss) on her mind. We wondered if Martin was naturally shy, or had been teased, or was unsuccessfully struggling to learn the skills of social communication, resulting in his isolation. We considered whether Curtis was feeling insecure about his new school, or if he had difficulty managing stress or ambiguity, or whether he operated under rigid thought systems that left him with few options to consider (feeling sure that a half-heard comment was an insult or that he could not apologize to a new acquaintance).

We learned that we are not likely to know the reasons for children's distress unless we give them an opportunity and a safe environment for them to express themselves freely. It goes without saying that if at any time we have reason to believe that a child should come to the attention of a professional counselor, a referral must be made, as had transpired with Fatima. A proactive referral system will be discussed at the end of this chapter. The upcoming section will describe a sampling of materials available for nonprofessional counselors to help children with developing a more positive self-concept and more satisfying social skills.

Why Provide Intervention?

When children are experiencing the kinds of difficulties described in this book, it is naive to believe that "things will work themselves out" or that "all children learn how to make friends eventually." Loeb and Sarigiani (1986) showed that children with hearing loss seemed to perceive their communication barriers as virtually insurmountable, and that they showed little belief in their ability to change themselves. Asher and his colleagues have studied "rejected and neglected children" for years (for example, Asher & Coie, 1990; Asher & Gottman, 1981), and have determined that for a variety of reasons, prosocial behaviors elude some children, but they can be taught these with directed coaching (Bierman & Furman, 1984). For example, preschoolers with hearing loss have been taught a set of simple social skills which resulted in a reduction in the amount of solitary and parallel play. These skills were still being used a year later (Antia & Kreimeyer, 1997).

Completing the counseling process may require more programmatic support than a counseling conversation as depicted in our scenarios. Following are suggestions for a range of interventions.

"Friendship Coaching"

Oden and Asher (1977) describe a program that can be adapted by most professionals for most environments. It does not require special materials per se, just a directed set of instructions on social skills with guided practice in safe environments.

They used a "coaching" approach to teach social skills necessary for friendship development. Over the course of four weeks, children identified as having few friends received several 5–7 minute mini-lessons on these four concepts:

- Participation (getting started in a game or activity, paying attention)
- Cooperation (taking turns, sharing)
- Communication (talking and listening to other children)
- Validation support, or "being friendly, fun, and nice" (looking at other children, giving a smile, offering help or encouragement)

In the first few sessions, the adult "coach" taught each concept and explained why they were important (for example, why cooperation made a game more fun), and then checked for understanding by asking children for examples of these concepts as well as opposite behaviors. The coach asked children to evaluate which behaviors would make activities enjoyable for everyone playing, and then asked children to try out some of the ideas in a follow-up play session (playing Pick-Up sticks, for example). Afterward, children had a 3–5 minute post-play review to evaluate which ideas were most helpful to make activities fun.

When children mastered all the concepts both cognitively and behaviorally, the coach expanded the instruction to classroom activities: "What are some of the games or activities you could play in the classroom or at recess with other kids?" Children were asked to generate ideas and try them out as a way of generalizing their new skills (participate, cooperate, communicate, validate): that is, to think of alternative suggestions and compromises (rather than fighting) if they disagreed about rules; to remember to talk with and ask questions about the other child while they play; to listen to and look at the other child to see how he or she is doing; to say something nice when the other person does well; to smile and offer help or suggestions and encouragement.

To determine the effectiveness of this coaching technique, the authors coached 12 third- and fourth-graders identified as the least liked in their classes. To avoid stigma, the children were told they were acting as "consultants" to the coach, who was trying to learn what kinds of things make it more enjoyable to play games. This coaching approach had a very positive outcome: not only did sociometric ratings improve immediately after training, but a year later they were still in the middle of classroom popularity.

"Friendship coaching" is a simple, direct, and effective way to provide personal adjustment support. Schum (1994) used the same approach in teaching social skills as well. While using any age-appropriate activity, he described how adults can directly teach or coach social skills:

1. Use modeling, by demonstrating how to do something with a clear example (how to order from a menu, how to act at a funeral or at a birthday party).
2. Rehearse, and provide specific feedback.
3. Preview the real activity. Discuss what will probably happen and how to respond.
4. Provide side-by-side support. An adult can be a "shadow" and provide on-line cues about what to do and say.
5. Check for comprehension, both after the preview and after the actual activity.

Following are additional resources designed to promote a positive self-concept, communication skills, and social problem-solving strategies. The first set of resources are for professionals, followed by a set of recommended reading materials for parents.

Resources for Professionals

1. Curriculum: *The PATHS Curriculum* by Kusche & Greenberg (1993).

PATHS stands for "**P**romoting **A**lternative **T**hinking **S**trategies," which will remind the reader of the REBT approach described in Chapter 3. This curriculum was developed first for children with hearing impairment and was later adapted for children without hearing impairment as well. It is a comprehensive set of lessons and activities (five volumes plus instructor's manual and other materials) designed to teach self-control, affective awareness, and social problem-solving skills, including problem identification, anger management, and goal setting. Lessons are developmentally appropriate for children from kindergarten though sixth grade. Students are given abundant opportunity for self-expression, promoting self-awareness and self-acceptance.

The material is intended to reflect a pervasive "classroom culture" of respect and regard for others. Research has shown this curriculum to be highly effective in helping children develop linguistic and cognitive control over impulsive behavior, increase their understanding of their emotions, and improve their interpersonal problem-solving skills (Greenburg & Kusche, 1993). A two-day training program is available for teachers and others.

>Available from: Developmental Research and Programs
>800/736-2630
><http://www.drp.org/PATHS/PATHS.html>

2.   Curriculum: *Knowledge is Power (KIP): A Program to Help Students Learn About Their Hearing Loss*, by Martilla and Mills (1994).

This curriculum was first developed in 1989 and is currently in its third edition. It is designed specifically for children who are deaf and hard of hearing, with the program goal of helping students "understand their hearing loss and its ramifications as completely as possible so they do not view themselves as handicapped." As a binder of more than 500 pages, it contains 12 sections on topics such as hearing anatomy, hearing tests, and hearing aids. It also includes sections on "Coping With a Hearing Loss," which poses questions for discussion such as:

- Will you have a hearing loss when you grow up?
- Does your family accept your hearing loss?
- Whom do you talk to when you have a problem?
- Can your thoughts and beliefs about hearing loss discourage your participation in school activities?

A unit on "Nurturing Friendships" is included in this section. An additional section on "Rational Emotive Education" is provided to help students understand that "no one is perfect" and to identify and change thoughts and beliefs about hearing loss and hearing aids that are not helpful to them. This curriculum is flexible and can be easily individualized to any educational setting.

>Available from: Mississippi Bend Area Educational Agency
>800/947-2329

3.   Materials: The "Skillstreaming" Series by Goldstein and McGinnis.

■ *Skillstreaming the Elementary School Child* (Rev. Ed.), book (339 pages) and skill cards (480 count). Target audience: Grades 1–5
■ *Skillstreaming the Adolescent* (Rev. Ed.), book (337 pages) and skill cards (400 count). Target audience: Grades 6–12

Each program teaches 50–60 skill steps toward developing prosocial behaviors. The books describe modeling techniques, role-playing activities, and methods to provide feedback and transfer training. The cards are used for group work, and list behavioral steps for each social skill.
    Social skills are divided into five areas:

■ Classroom Survival Skills (listening, asking a question, ignoring distractions, setting a goal)
■ Friendship-Making Skills (introducing oneself, beginning/ending a conversation, joining in, sharing, apologizing)
■ Skills for Dealing with Feelings (knowing/expressing one's feelings, recognizing another's feelings, expressing concern and affection, dealing with fear)
■ Skill Alternatives to Aggression (asking permission, responding to teasing, staying out of fights, accepting consequences, negotiating)
■ Skills for Dealing with Stress (dealing with boredom, losing, and group pressure, making a complaint, reacting to failure)

The original versions were published in 1984 and were brought back into print because of the high demand. It is considered a classic resource. Although not designed specifically for children with hearing loss, the materials are readily adaptable.

    Available from: Thinking Publications
                       800/225-GROW
                       <http://www.ThinkingPublications.com>

4.   Handbook: *Let's Converse: A "How-To" Guide to Develop and Expand Conversational Skills of Children and Teenagers Who Are Hearing Impaired*, by Nancy Tye-Murray (1994).

This 233-page guide covers questions such as "What are conversational rules?" and ties them directly to hearing loss. She provides many do's and don'ts, such as providing sufficient time for a child to express her thoughts. Communication breakdowns and repair strategies are described throughout, with an ongoing theme of children learning how to be assertive when they do not understand. A particularly relevant chapter is entitled, "Requisites for Conversation: Engendering Social Skills," which describes how social skills are learned through both observation and direct instruction, and how hearing loss can inhibit the development of social maturity. Step-by-step instructions are provided to help adults teach essential social skills. Many activities and exercises are described in the appendices. The book is written for the general reader and can be quickly adapted to most social settings, particularly school.

Available from:	Alexander Graham Bell Association
	202/337-5220 (voice); 202/337-5221 (TTY)
	<http://www.agbell.org>

5.   Video: *Emotional intelligence: The key to social skills*
This 29-minute video is designed for professionals who want to learn innovative teaching techniques in helping children social skills such as how to listen, share, and be kind. Psychologist Daniel Goleman discusses the nature of emotional intelligence and how it develops; child psychologist Maurice Elias explains emotional literacy.

Available from:	Films for the Humanities and Sciences
	800-257-5126
	<http://www.films.com>

Resources for Parents

Following is a brief list of reading materials recommended to parents interested in helping their child develop a more positive self-concept and in developing more productive communication on affective issues. None are written with deaf or hard-of-hearing children in mind, but the points made are applicable to all families. Ginott's books are classics in parenting literature, and most of the others are based on his recommendations. These books can be found in most local libraries.

- Apter, T. (1997). *The confident child: Raising children to believe in themselves*. New York: Bantam Books.
- Denkin, E. (2000). *Why can't you catch me being good?* Holbrook, MA: Adams Media.

- Elias, M., Tobias, S., & Friedlander, B. (1999). *Emotionally intelligent parenting: How to raise a self-disciplined, responsible, socially skilled child.* New York: Three Rivers Press.
- Faber, A., & Mazlish, E. (1980). *How to talk so kids will listen and how to listen so kids will talk.* New York: Avon Books.
- Ginott, H. (1965). *Between parent and child.* New York: Macmillan.
- Ginott, H. (1969). *Between parent and teen.* New York: Macmillan.
- Glenn, S. & Nelson, J. (2000). *Raising self-reliant children in a self-indulgent world (revised).* Rocklin, CA: Prima Publishing Communications.
- Marano, H., E. (1988). *"Why doesn't anyone like me?" A guide to raising socially confident kids.* New York: William Morrow.

Referring to Professional Counselors

There is no magic formula to advise us when a referral to a professional counselor is in order, but as one becomes familiar with the content covered in this book, and with any of the materials described above, it is probable we can almost immediately determine our boundaries. The wisest "rule of thumb" is: *when in doubt, refer.* When we even begin to wonder if a child is experiencing stress that he or she cannot manage, or has dysfunctional components in his or her life, the time to refer is NOW.

Four steps are needed in the development of a referral system:

1. Be proactive
2. Collaborate on referral sources
3. Document
4. Follow up

Be Proactive

Professionals are exhorted to have a predeveloped referral process in place, and to organize contact information before a crisis arises. The following template is provided as a generic framework from which to organize information. It is acknowledged that each community will have its own resources from which to draw on. Referrals for children and families may or may not overlap. The point is to keep such information foremost in one's system, and make use of it in a proactive rather than a reactive way:

When concerned about a child:

Agency	Contact Person	Phone/pager number

When concerned about parents/family:

Agency	Contact Person	Phone/pager number

Collaborate on Referral Sources

It is recommended that this information be collected from all individuals associated with a program, rather than depending on one person to be aware of all community resources. It is quite common for some colleagues to have only some of the information available, and a core or collective referral system should have input from all parties. Procedures for contact should be agreed on by all members of the program; for example, confidentiality must be respected, and a program must decide whether electronic communication (E-mail) is secure enough.

Documentation and Follow-Up

At the very least, each telephone or face-to-face contact must be documented by writing down a summary of the conversation, with a date and a signature or initial. Copies of written reports need to be authorized by signed release forms. Follow-up procedures should be established to ensure that a contact person is aware of the status of the referral. No assumption should be made that a referral is being carried out as intended.

Chapter Summary

- Children can be effectively guided to find solutions to their problems by helping them identify goals and then implement plans to reach their goals. The more they take the lead in this process, the more problem-solving skills they acquire.
- Children will demonstrate individual differences in problem-solving based on prior experience as well as their personality and the situation they face.
- The expectation or hope that children will outgrow their difficulties or "figure them out" on their own cannot be perpetuated.
- This chapter provided a set of resources for professionals and parents who desire to provide social and affective intervention for children with hearing loss.
- It is hoped that the information presented in this book will convey urgency and provide direction to professionals and parents as they consider all the needs of children growing up with hearing loss.

Learning Activities

Clarification Activity

Describe to a learning partner why Fatima's teacher did not get further involved in the counseling process.

Modeling Activity

With a learning partner, interview a school counselor or other professional counselor, and ask how he or she would work with this problem expressed by Sam, who is 16 and hard of hearing:

"I was thinking about applying for a job at the stadium, but I don't think the people there would understand me when I talk to them."

Ask the professional counselor to describe an overall strategy to help Sam.

Writing Activity

Write a few paragraphs summarizing what you learned from the professional counselor.

Practice/Feedback

With a learning partner, develop a skit reflecting the strategies learned from your interview, and present, this a group for feedback. Did the "counselor" help "Sam" to solve his own problem or did the counselor solve it for him?

Suggested Readings

Meyers, L. H., Park, H. S., Grenot-Scheyer, M., Schwartz, I. S., & Harry, B. (1998). *Making friends: The influence of culture and development*. Baltimore: Paul H. Brooks.

This 456-page book describes the process of friendship development in young children. Research models describe the effects of disability as well as other diversities on the social relationships of children, and strategies are provided to help the interventionist promote respect and sensitivity in the environment while turning problematic behaviors into prosocial ones. Hearing loss is not mentioned specifically, although disability in general is. The information in this book would be helpful for those interested in exploring friendship development as part of a research program or project.

Schloss, P. J., & Smith, M. (1990*). Teaching social skills to hearing impaired students*. Washington, DC: Alexander Graham Bell Association.

This book (203 pages) provides a framework for teaching and modifying social behavior in children with hearing losses (all ages). The authors describe how to identify skill priorities, goals and objectives, and develop instructional activities. Games, learning centers, and homework activities are provided.

CHAPTER 6

Self-Evaluation: How Am I Doing As a Counselor?

Any new skill warrants evaluation, and counseling is no exception. Just as the children we are counseling are encouraged to evaluate their action plans, so should we also consider our own "learning curve" and be mindful of where we still need to improve.

The most obvious way to determine if one's counseling skills are effective is to look for a positive change in a child's behavior. It would be hoped that, as a result of nonprofessional counseling efforts, Fatima would no longer be withdrawn, begin to regain her lost weight, and feel generally happier; that Martin would develop social skills to help with friendship development; that Curtis would resolve his misunderstanding with his teammate and maintain his membership on the track team. If at any time it appears that a child is still struggling, it is not to be considered a failure in nonprofessional counseling, but rather an even clearer sign that a referral to a professional counselor is in order. Nonprofessional counseling is one of the strands of the "safety net" mentioned in Chapter 1, but it is not intended to replace the essential support provided by professional counselors.

Following is an informal "self-evaluation quiz," that is, a set of statements designed to help the reader conduct an evaluation of his or her growth in counseling abilities. It is hoped that the reader will review these items more than once, and focus on improving one skill at a time, rather than attempting to be "super-counselor" immediately. Please note that there are no number values to the answers and no percentages designated as "superior," "fair," or "poor." It is recommended that the counselor-in-training complete the quiz now, and then return to it in two weeks, after concerted effort to improve on one skill. If you feel that you have improved, then another skill can be targeted, and so on.

Growing As a Counselor: Self-Evaluation Quiz

1. I can differentiate between a request for information and a personal adjustment comment.

   usually   am improving   room for growth

2. I refrain from giving information when presented with a personal adjustment comment.

   usually   am improving   room for growth

3. I recognize when a "communication mismatch" has occurred.

   usually   am improving   room for growth

4. I understand the difference between professional and nonprofessional counseling.

   usually   am improving   room for growth

5. I can describe the cyclical nature of the development of self-concept.

   usually   am improving   room for growth

6. I can perceive the "hearing aid effect" from a child's point of view.

   usually   am improving   room for growth

7. I can appreciate the "hearing aid effect" from a parent's point of view.

   usually   am improving   room for growth

8. I can explain the concepts of congruence and unconditional positive regard.

   usually   am improving   room for growth

9. I can describe conditions in which the REBT approach would be helpful.

   usually   am improving   room for growth

10. I can competently administer a "door-opening" activity (e.g., *CPR Scale, I Start/You Finish, Readiness Scale*).

    usually   am improving   room for growth

11. I actively monitor the amount of "talk time" I use.

    usually   am improving   room for growth

12. I do not dispense advice when a child is figuring out his or her problem.

    usually   am improving   room for growth

13. I see the child as the "expert" of his or her own life.

    usually   am improving   room for growth

14. I do not "grab the conversational controls," but give that control to the child.

    usually   am improving   room for growth

15. I know what is meant by the question, "Who owns this hearing loss?"

    usually   am improving   room for growth

16. I use minimal encouragers and paraphrasing frequently.

    usually   am improving   room for growth

17. I am comfortable in reflecting/acknowledging feelings.

    usually   am improving   room for growth

18. I give feedback, when it is solicited, in descriptive and specific words.

    usually   am improving   room for growth

19. I use silence as a counseling tool.

    usually   am improving   room for growth

20. I can explain why reassurance can actually make a person feel worse, not better.

    usually   am improving   room for growth

22. I can recognize habituation when it occurs.

    usually   am improving   room for growth

23. I am able to refrain from "identifying" ("That happened to me!") at the wrong moment.

    usually   am improving   room for growth

24. During counseling conversations, I am listening more and talking less often than I used to.

    usually   am improving   room for growth

25. I can guide a child through the process of setting goals and developing plans without "taking over."

    usually   am improving   room for growth

REFERENCES

Altman, E. (1996). Meeting the needs of adolescents with impaired hearing. In F. Martin & J. G. Clark (Eds.), *Hearing care for children*, 197–210. Needham Heights, MA: Allyn & Bacon.

American Association for Counseling and Development. (1982). *Reflections with Carl Rogers: Great minds in counseling historical video series.* New York: Author.

Anderson, K. & Smaldino, J. (1998). *Learning Inventories for Education (LIFE).* Available from Educational Audiology Association, 4319 Ehrlich Road, Tampa FL 33624, 800/460-7322, <http://www.edaud.org.>

Anderson, K. & Smaldino, J. (2000). *Child Home Inventory of Listening Difficulties (CHILD).* Available from Educational Audiology Association, 4319 Ehrlich Road, Tampa FL 33624, 800/460-7322, <http://www.edaud.org.>

Antia, S. & Kreimeyer, K. (1992). Social competence intervention for young children with hearing impairments. In S. Odom, S. McConnell, & M. McEvoy (Eds.), *Social competence of young children with disabilities: Issues and strategies for intervention*, (135–64). Baltimore: Paul H. Brookes Publishing Co.

Antia, S. & Kreimeyer, K. (1997). The generalization and maintenance of the peer social behaviors of young children who are deaf or hard of hearing. *Language, Speech, and Hearing Services in Schools, 28,* 59–69

Asher, S. & Coie, D. (Eds.) (1990). *Peer rejection in childhood.* Cambridge: Cambridge University Press.

Asher, S. & Gottman, J. (Eds.). (1981). *The development of children's friendships.* Cambridge: Cambridge University Press.

Atkins, D. (1994) Counseling children with hearing loss and their families. In J. G. Clark & F. N. Martin (Eds.), *Effective counseling in audiology*, 116–46. Needham Heights: Allyn & Bacon.

Bachara, G., Raphael, J., & Phelan, W. (1980). Empathy development in deaf preadolescents. *American Annals of the Deaf, 125,* 38–41.

Beazley, S. & Moore, M. (1995). *Deaf children, their families, and professionals: Dismantling barriers.* London: David Fulton Publishers.

Bess, F. H., Dodd-Murphy, J., & Parker, R. (1998). Children with minimal sensorineural hearing loss: Prevalence, educational performance, and functional status. *Ear and Hearing, 19*(5), 339–55.

Bierman, L. L. & Furman, W. (1984). The effects of social skills training and peer involvement on the social adjustment of preadolescents. *Child Development, 55,* 151–62.

Blood, G. W., Blood, M., & Danhauer, J. L. (1977). The hearing aid "effect." *Hearing Instruments, 20,* 12.

Branthwaite, A. (1985). The development of social identity and self-concept. In A. Branthwaite & D. Rogers (Eds.), *Children growing up*, 34–42. Philadelphia: Open University Press.

Brimacombe, J. A., Danhauer, J. L., & Mulac, A. (1983). Teachers' perceptions of students who wear hearing aids: An empirical test. *Language, Speech, and Hearing Services in Schools, 14,* 128–35.

Byrne, B. M. (1996). *Measuring self-concept across the lifespan.* Washington, DC: American Psychology Association.

Calderon, R. & Greenberg, M. (1999). Stress and coping in hearing mothers of children with hearing loss: Factors affecting mother and child adjustment. *American Annals of the Deaf, 144*(1).

Cappelli, M., Daniels, T., Durleux-Smith, A., McGrath, P. J., & Neuss, D. (1995). Social development of children with hearing impairments who are integrated into general education classrooms. *Volta Review, 97,* 197–208.

Clark, J. G. (1994). Audiologists' counseling purview. In J. G. Clark & F. N. Martin (Eds.), *Effective counseling in audiology: Perspectives and practices,* 1–17. Englewood Cliffs, NJ: Prentice Hall.

Clark, J. G. (1999). Working with challenging patients. *Audiology Today, 11*(5), 13–15.

Cohen, O. P. (1978). The deaf adolescent: Who am I? *Volta Review, 80,* 265–70.

Combes, A. W. & Gonzales, D. M. (1994*). Helping relationships: Basic concepts for the helping professions* (4th ed.). Boston, MA: Allyn & Bacon.

Cormier, S. & Hackney, H. (1999). *Counseling strategies and interventions* (5th ed.). Boston: Allyn & Bacon.

Coyner, L. (1993). Academic success, self-concept, social acceptance, and perceived social acceptance for hearing, hard of hearing, and deaf students in a mainstream setting. *Journal of the American Deafness and Rehabilitation Association, 27*(2), 13–20.

Crowe, T. (1997a). Approaches to counseling. In T. Crowe (Ed.), *Applications in counseling in speech-language pathology and audiology,* 80–117. Baltimore, MD: Williams and Wilkins.

Crowe, T. (1997b). Counseling: Definition, history, rationale. In T. Crowe (Ed.), *Applications in counseling in speech-language pathology and audiology,* 2–29. Baltimore, MD: Williams and Wilkins.

Culpepper, B., Mendel, L. L., & McCarthy, P. A. (1994). Counseling experience and training offered by ESB-accredited programs. *Asha, 36*(6), 55–58.

Davis, J., Elfenbein, J., Schum, R., & Bentler, R. (1986). Effects of mild and moderate hearing impairments on language, educational, and psychosocial behavior of children. *Journal of Speech and Hearing Disorders, 51,* 53–62.

Dengerink, J. E. & Porter, J. B. (1984). Children's attitudes toward peers wearing hearing aids. *Language, Speech, and Hearing Services in Schools, 15,* 205–08.

Doggett, S., Stein, R., & Gans, D. (1998). Hearing aid effect in older females. *Journal of American Academy of Audiology, 9*(5), 361–66.

Edwards, C. (1991). The transition from auditory training to holistic auditory management. *Educational Audiology Monograph, 2,* 1–17.

Egan, G. (1998). *The skilled helper* (6th ed.). Pacific Grove, CA: Brooks/Cole.

Ellis, A. (1962). *Reason and emotion in psychotherapy.* Secaucus, NJ: Lyle Stuart.

English, K. (1997). *Self-advocacy for students who are deaf and hard of hearing.* Austin, TX: Pro-Ed.

English, K. (2001, April). Peer relationships: Teachers' and children's perceptions. Paper presented at the American Academy of Audiology Conference, San Diego, CA.

English, K., Mendel, L. L., Rojeski, T., & Hornak, J. (1999). Counseling in audiology, or learning to listen: Pre- and post-measures from an audiology counseling course. *American Journal of Audiology, 8*(1), 34–39.

English, K., Rojeski, T., & Branham, K. (2000). Acquiring counseling skills in mid-career: Outcomes of a distance education course for practicing audiologists. *Journal of the American Academy of Audiology, 11*, 84–90.

Faber, A. & Mazlish, E. (1995). *How to talk so kids can learn.* New York: Simon and Schuster.

Flexer, C. (1999). *Facilitating hearing and listening in young children* (2d ed). San Diego: Singular Publishing Group.

Gange, R. M. (1980). Learnable aspects of problem solving. *Educational Psychologist, 15*, 84–92.

Ginott, H. (1969). *Between parent and teenager.* New York: MacMillan Co.

Giolas, T. G., Maxon, A. B., & Kessler, A. B. (1997). *Hearing Performance Inventory for Children (HPIC).* Available from Educational Audiology Association, 4319 Ehrlich Road, Tampa FL 33624, 800/460–7322, <http://www.edaud.org>.

Goleman, D. (1995). *Emotional intelligence: Why it can matter more than IQ.* New York: Bantam Books.

Greenberg, M. T. & Kusche, C. A. (1993). *Promoting social and emotional development in deaf children: The PATHS project.* Seattle: University of Washington Press.

Gresham, F. M. & Elliot, S. N. (1990). *Social skills rating system.* Circle Pines, MI: American Guidance Service.

Grunblatt, H. & Daar, L. (1994). A support program: Audiological counseling. *Language, Speech, and Hearing Services in Schools, 25*, 112–14.

Haley, D. J. & Hood, S. B. (1986). Young adolescents' perception of their peers who wear hearing aids. *Journal of Communicative Disorders, 19*, 449–60.

Harris, L. K., Van Zandt, C. E., & Rees, T. H. (1997). Counseling needs of students who are deaf and hard of hearing. *The School Counselor, 44*, 271–79.

Hartup, W. W. (1996). The company they keep: Friendships and their developmental significance. *Child Development, 67*, 1–13.

Henggeler, S. W., Watson, S. M., & Whelan, J. P. (1990). Peer relations of hearing-impaired adolescents. *Journal of Pediatric Psychology, 15*(6), 721–31.

Jamieson, J. R. (1995). Interactions between mothers and children who are deaf. *Journal of Early Intervention, 19*(2), 108–17.

Kelly, L. J. (1992). Rational-emotive therapy and aural rehabilitation. *Journal of the Academy of Rehabilitative Audiology, 25*, 43–50.

Kennedy, E. & Charles, S. (1989). *On becoming a counselor: A basic guide for nonprofessional counselors.* New York: Consortium.

Kimmel, D. C. & Weiner, I. B. (1995). *Adolescence: A developmental transition.* New York: Wiley and Sons.

Kricos, P. B. (2000). Family counseling for children with hearing loss. In J. Alpiner & P. A. McCarthy (Eds.), *Rehabilitative audiology: Children and adults* (3d ed.), 275–302. Philadelphia: Lipincot Williams & Wilkins.

Kroth, R. L. (1987). Mixed or missed messages between parents and professionals. *Volta Review, 89*, 1–10.

Kusche, A. A., Garfield, T. S., & Greenberg, M. T. (1983). The understanding of emotional and social attributions in deaf adolescents. *Journal of Clinical Child Psychology, 12*, 153–60.

Lapore, S. J. (1997). Social-environmental influences on the chronic state process. In B. H. Gottlieb (Ed.), *Coping with chronic stress*, 133–60. New York: Plenum Press.

Loeb, R. & Sarigiani, P. (1986). The impact of hearing impairment on self-perceptions of children. *Volta Review, 86*, 89–100.

Long, V. O. (1996). *Communication skills in helping relationships*. Pacific Grove, CA: Brookes/Cole.

Lundberg, G. & Lundberg, J. (1995). *"I don't have to make it all better": Six practical principles that empower others to solve their own problems while enriching your relationship*. New York: Penguin Books.

Luterman, D. (1995). Counseling of parents of children with auditory disorders. In R. J. Roesser & M. Downs (Eds.), *Auditory disorders in children*, 353–61. NY: Thieme.

Luterman, D. L. (1996). *Counseling persons with communication disorders and their families* (3d ed.). Austin, TX: Pro-Ed.

Marsh, H. (1992). *Self Description Questionnaire II (SDQ II)*. Available from the School of Education and Language Studies, University of Western Sydney, PO Box 555, Campbell, New South Wales 2650, Australia.

Martin, F. N., George, K. A., O'Neal, J., & Daly, J. A. (1987). Audiologists' and parents' attitudes regarding counseling of families of hearing impaired children. *Asha, 29*(2), 27–33.

Marttila, J. & Mills, M. (1994). *Knowledge is power*. Available from Mississippi Bend Area Education Agency, Special Education Division, 729 21st Street, Bettendorf, IA, 52722-5096, 800-947-2329.

Maxon, A., Brackett, D., & van den Berg. (1991). Self-perception of socialization: The effects of hearing status, age, and gender. *Volta Review, 93*(1), 7–18.

McCarthy, P., Culpepper, B., & Lucks, L. (1986). Variability in counseling experiences and training among ESB-accredited programs. *Asha, 28*(9), 49–52.

McCay, V. (1996). Psychosocial aspects of hearing impairment. In R. Schow & M. Nerbonne (Eds.), *Introduction to audiologic rehabilitation* (3d ed., 229–63). Needham Heights, MA: Allyn & Bacon.

McGinnis, E. & Goldstein, A. P. (1984). *Skillstreaming the elementary school child: A guide for teaching prosocial skills*. Champaign, IL: Research Press Co.

Meadow, K. (1976). Personality and social development of deaf persons. *Journal of Rehabilitation of the Deaf, 9*, 3–16.

Meadow, K. (1980). *Deafness and child development*. Berkeley, CA: University of California Press.

Meadow-Orlans, K. P. (1983). *Meadow-Kendall social-emotional assessment inventories for deaf and hearing-impaired students*. Washington, DC: Gallaudet University Outreach Pre-College Program.

Mendel, L. L. (1997). Children and adolescents with hearing impairment and their parents. In T. Crow (Ed.), *Applications of counseling in speech-language pathology and audiology*, 290–306. Baltimore: Williams and Wilkins.

Murphy, L. O. & Ross, S. M. (1987). Gender differences in the social problem-solving performance of adolescents. *Sex Roles, 16,* (5–6), 251–64.

Nelson, E., Wasson, J., Kirk, J., Keller, A., Clark, D., Deitrich, A., Stewart, A., & Zubkoff, M. (1987). Assessment of function in routine clinical practice: Description of the COOP Chart Method and preliminary findings. *Journal of Chronic Disability, 40* (Suppl. 1), 555–635.

Oden, S. & Asher, S. (1977). Coaching children in social skills for friendship making. *Child Development, 48,* 495–506.

Palmer, C., Butts, S., Lindley, G., & Snyder, S. (1996). *Time out! I didn't hear you.* Pittsburgh, PA: Sports Support Syndicate. Also available online: <http://www.pitt.edu/~commsci/pubs/timeout.pdf>

Palmer, C. & Mormer, E. (1998). Defining the child's and parent's expectations of the hearing aid fitting. *Hearing Journal, 51*(9), 80.

Palmer, P. J. (1998). *The courage to teach.* San Francisco: Jossey-Bass.

Parsons, R. D. (1995). *The skills of helping.* Boston: Allyn & Bacon.

Piers, E. V. (1984). *Piers-Harris Children's Self-Concept Scale-Revised.* (1984). Available from Western Psychological Services, 12031 Wilshire Blvd, Los Angeles CA 90025-1251.

Piers, E. V. & Harris, D. B. (1964). Age and other correlates of self- concept in children. *Journal of Educational Psychology, 55,* 91–95.

Pipp-Siegel, S. & Biringen, Z. (2000). Assessing the quality of relationships between parents and children: The Emotional Availability Scales. *Volta Review, 100*(5)(monograph), 237–49.

Pudlas, K. (1996). Self-esteem and self-concept: Special education as experienced by deaf, hard of hearing, and hearing students. *British Columbia Journal of Special Education, 20*(1), 23–39.

Purkey, W. (1984). *Inviting school success: A self-concept approach to teaching and learning.* Belmont, CA: Wadsworth Publishing Co.

Raymond, K. L. & Matson, J. L. (1989). Social skills in the hearing impaired. *Journal of Clinical Child Psychology, 18*(3), 247–58.

Reik, T. (1949). *Listening with the third ear.* New York: Farrar, Strauss.

Reinsche, L. L., Peterson, K. J., & Linden, S. L. (1990). Young children's attitudes toward peer hearing aid wearers. *Hearing Journal, 43*(10), 19–20.

Rogers, C. (1961). *On becoming a person.* Boston: Houghton-Mifflin.

Rogers, C. (1986). Client centered therapy. In I. L. Kutash & A. Wolf (Eds.), *Psychotherapist's casebook: Therapy and technique in practice.* San Francisco: Jossey-Bass.

Ronning, R. R., McCurdy, D., & Ballinger, R. (1984). Individual differences: A third component in problem-solving instruction. *Journal of Research in Science Teaching, 21*(1), 71–82.

Rotter Incomplete Sentences Blank (2d ed.) (1992). Available from the Psychological Corporation, 555 Academic Ct., San Antonio TX 78204-2498.

Rumberger, R. (1995). Dropping out of middle school: A multilevel analysis of schools and students. *American Education Research Journal, 32,* 583–625.

Sanders, D. A. (1993). *Management of hearing handicap: Infants to elderly* (3d ed.). Englewood Cliffs, NJ: Prentice Hall.

Schum, R. (1991). Communication and social growth: A developmental model of social behavior in deaf children. *Ear and Hearing, 12*(5), 320–27.

Schum, R. & Gfeller, K. (1994). Requisites for conversation: Engendering social skills. In N. Tye-Murray (Ed.), *Let's converse: A "how-to" guide to develop and expand conversational skills of children and teenagers who are hearing impaired,* 147–76. Washington, DC: A. B. Bell Association.

Shames, G. H. (2000). *Counseling the communicatively disabled and their families: A manual for clinicians.* Boston: Allyn & Bacon.

Shipley, K. (1997). *Interviewing and counseling in communication disorders: Principles and procedures.* Boston: Allyn & Bacon.

Skinner, B. F. (1938). *The behavior of organisms.* New York: Appleton-Century-Crofts.

Skinner, B. F. (1953). *Science and human behavior.* New York: Macmillan.

Stein, R., Gill, K., & Gans, D. (2000). Adolescents' attitudes toward their peers with hearing impairment. *Journal of Educational Audiology, 8,* 1–8.

Stinson, M. S., Whitmore, K., & Kluwin, T. N. (1996). Self-perceptions of social relationships in hearing-impaired adolescents. *Journal of Educational Psychology, 88*(1), 132–43.

Stone, D., Patton, B., & Heen, S. (1999). *Difficult conversations: How to discuss what matters most.* New York: Viking Press.

Stone, J. R. & Olswang, L. B. (1989). The hidden challenge in counseling. *Asha, 31,* 27–31.

Strein, W. (1993). Advances on academic self-concept: Implications for school psychology. *School Psychology Review, 22*(2), 273–284.

Turnbull, A. & Turnbull, H. (1990). *Families, professionals, and exceptionalities: A special partnership* (2d ed.). Columbus, OH: Charles E. Merrill.

Von Almen, P. & Blair, J. (1989). Informational counseling for school-aged hearing-impaired students. *Language, Speech, and Hearing Services in Schools, 20,* 31–40.

Warren, C. & Hasenstab, S. (1986). Self-concept of severely to profoundly hearing impaired children. *Volta Review, 88,* 289–96.

APPENDIX

Children's Peer Relationship (CPR) Scale

#1. School

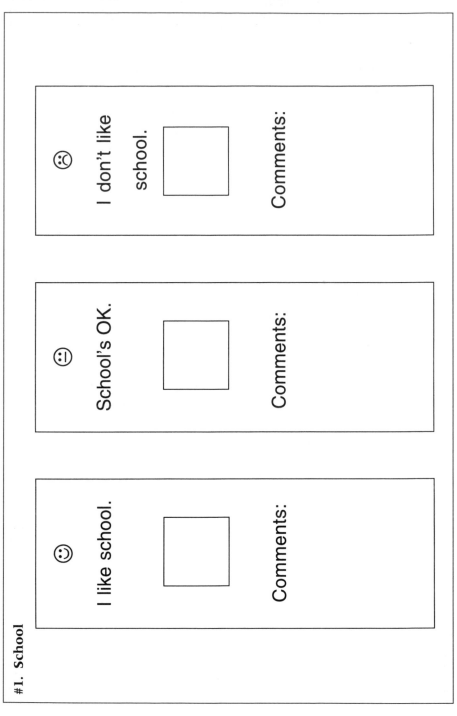

#2. Friends in School

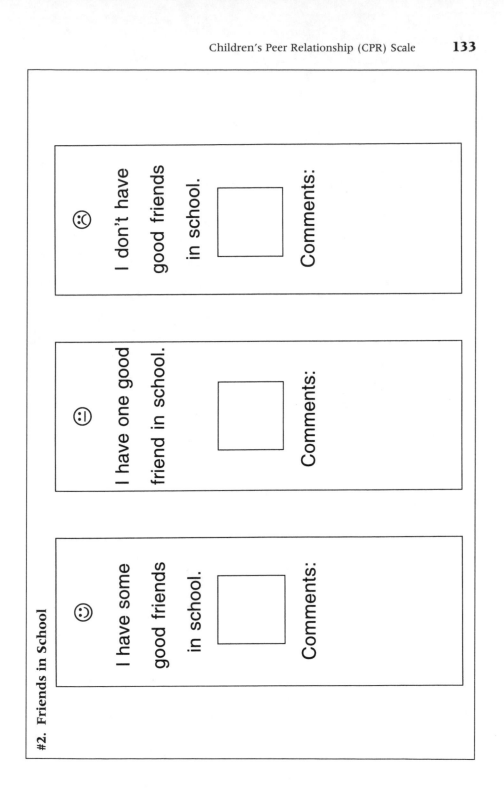

© I have some good friends in school.

Comments:

☺ I have one good friend in school.

Comments:

☹ I don't have good friends in school.

Comments:

#3. Best Friend

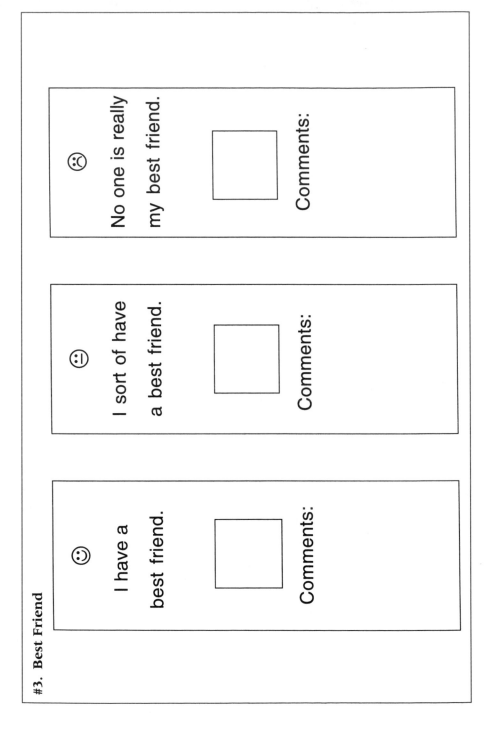

☺

I have a
best friend.

Comments:

☹

I sort of have
a best friend.

Comments:

☹

No one is really
my best friend.

Comments:

#4. Other Kids and Me

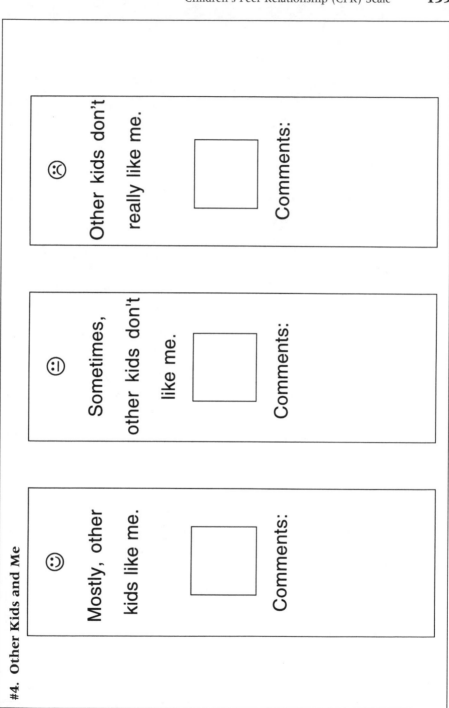

☺

Mostly, other kids like me.

Comments:

☺

Sometimes, other kids don't like me.

Comments:

☹

Other kids don't really like me.

Comments:

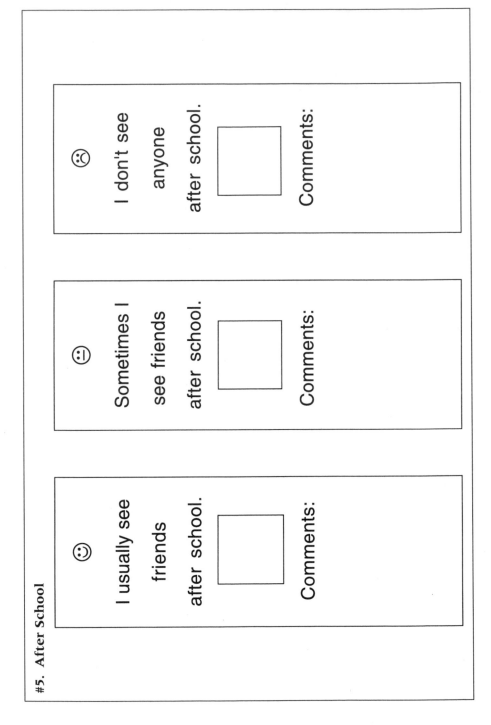

#5. After School

☺
I usually see
friends
after school.

Comments:

☺
Sometimes I
see friends
after school.

Comments:

☹
I don't see
anyone
after school.

Comments:

#6. Teasing

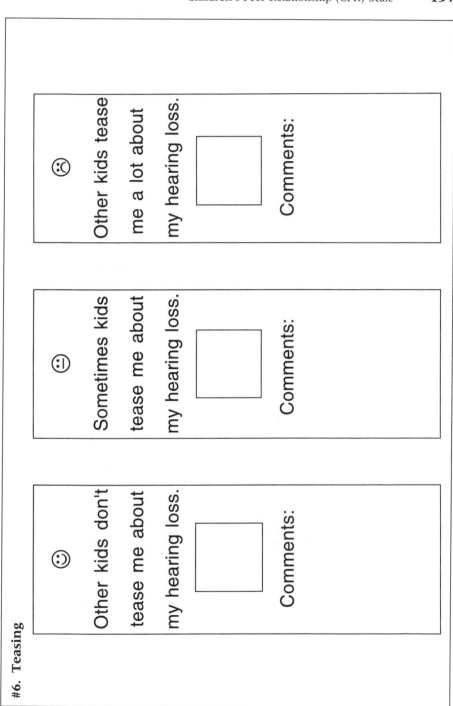

Other kids don't tease me about my hearing loss.

Comments:

Sometimes kids tease me about my hearing loss.

Comments:

Other kids tease me a lot about my hearing loss.

Comments:

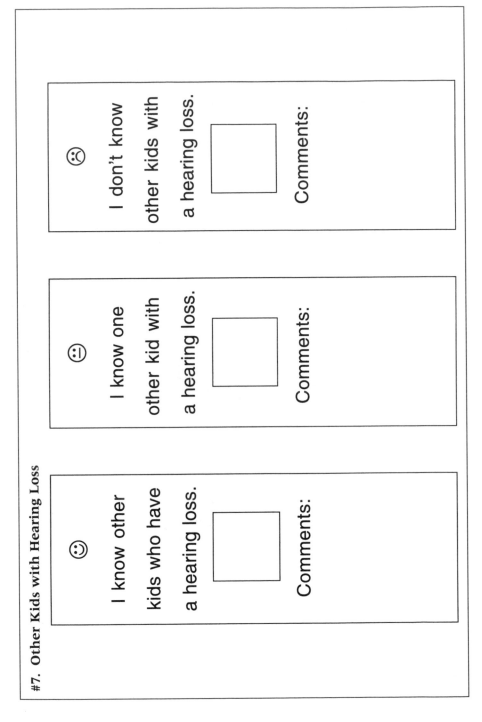

#7. Other Kids with Hearing Loss

☺

I know other
kids who have
a hearing loss.

Comments:

😐

I know one
other kid with
a hearing loss.

Comments:

☹

I don't know
other kids with
a hearing loss.

Comments:

#8/ha.   **What I Think about My Hearing Aids**

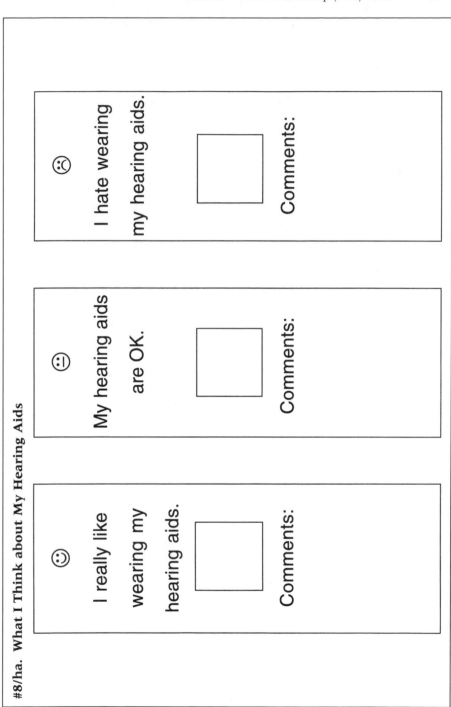

☺

I really like
wearing my
hearing aids.

Comments:

☺

My hearing aids
are OK.

Comments:

☹

I hate wearing
my hearing aids.

Comments:

#8/ci. What I Think about My Cochlear Implant

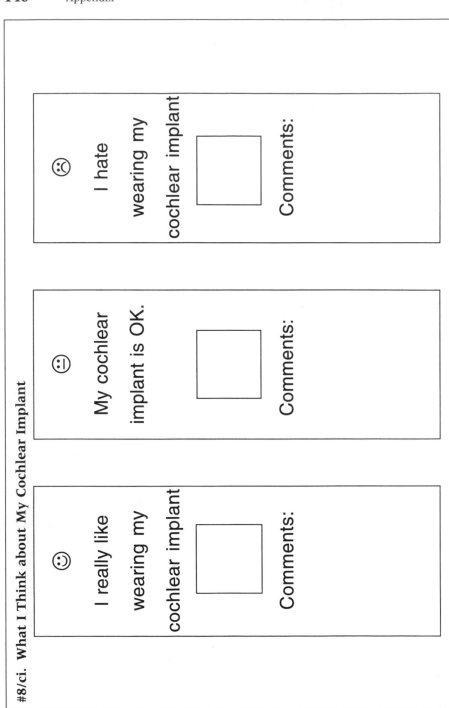

INDEX